Diabetic renal diet cookbook for beginners 2024

Culinary Solutions for Maintaining Healthy Blood Glucose and Kidney Performance

Ennis James

Copyright © 2024 by Ennis James

All rights reserved

No part of this publication may be reproduced, stored in a retrieval system, or transmitted, in any form or by any means, electronic, mechanical, photocopying, recording, or otherwise, without the prior written permission of the author.

The information in this ebook is true and complete to the best of our knowledge. All recommendation are made without guarantee on the part of author or publisher. The author and publisher disclaim any liability in connection with the use of this information.

Table of Contents

Introduction   4
- Understanding Diabetes and Kidney Disease   8
- Benefits of a Diabetic Renal Diet   11
- Essential Nutrients for Kidney Health   14
- Tips for Meal Planning and Preparation   17
- How to Use This Cookbook   20

Chapter 1: Breakfast Delights   23
- Spinach and Mushroom Omelette   23
- Blueberry Almond Overnight Oats   26
- Greek Yogurt with Fresh Berries and Chia Seeds   29
- Quinoa Breakfast Bowl with Apples and Cinnamon   31
- Scrambled Tofu with Vegetables   34
- Whole Grain Avocado Toast   37
- Berry and Spinach Smoothie   40
- Cottage Cheese with Pineapple   42
- Low-Sodium Turkey and Egg White Breakfast Wrap   44
- Spiced Apple and Oat Muffins   47

Chapter 2: Lunch Solutions   50
- Grilled Chicken Salad with Lemon Vinaigrette   50
- Lentil and Vegetable Soup   53
- Quinoa and Black Bean Salad   56
- Baked Cod with Steamed Broccoli   59
- Turkey and Spinach Wrap   61
- Chickpea and Avocado Sandwich   64

Roasted Vegetable and Hummus Bowl	67
Cauliflower Rice Stir-Fry	70
Mediterranean Tuna Salad	73
Zucchini Noodles with Pesto and Cherry Tomatoes	75
Chapter 3: Dinner Choices	**78**
Herb-Crusted Salmon with Asparagus	78
Stuffed Bell Peppers with Ground Turkey	81
Baked Chicken with Rosemary and Sweet Potatoes	84
Spinach and Ricotta Stuffed Portobello Mushrooms	87
Beef and Broccoli Stir-Fry	90
Lemon Garlic Shrimp with Quinoa	93
Eggplant Parmesan (Baked)	96
Grilled Tofu with Steamed Vegetables	99
Spaghetti Squash with Turkey Marinara	102
Vegetable and Lentil Stew	105
Chapter 4: Snacks and Sides	**108**
Cucumber and Hummus Bites	108
Baked Kale Chips	110
Conclusion	**112**

Introduction

In a quaint little town, nestled between rolling hills and lush greenery, lived a woman named Lisa. Lisa had always been the heart of her family, her warmth and love evident in the delicious meals she prepared every day. But life threw her a curveball when she was diagnosed with diabetes, and shortly after, kidney disease. The news was a heavy blow, and Lisa found herself overwhelmed with the complex dietary restrictions that came with managing both conditions.

One sunny afternoon, as she sat in her cozy kitchen, Lisa stared at her once-beloved recipe book, now filled with dishes she could no longer enjoy. Her husband, Mark, noticed the sadness in her eyes and wrapped his arms around her. "We'll figure this out together," he said softly. But deep down, Lisa knew they needed more than just determination—they needed guidance.

Weeks turned into months, and Lisa's health journey became increasingly challenging. The internet was flooded with conflicting information, and the local library's resources were outdated. Lisa needed a solution, something reliable and practical, to help her regain control over her health without losing the joy of cooking.

One day, a dear friend recommended a book that had transformed her own health: "Diabetic Renal Diet Cookbook for Beginners 2024." Intrigued, Lisa immediately ordered a copy. When it arrived, she was struck by the vibrant cover and the promise of a new beginning. As she flipped through the pages, hope started to blossom within her.

The introduction was warm and welcoming, explaining the basics of diabetes and kidney disease in simple terms. It was like having a conversation with a caring friend who understood her struggles. The book emphasized the importance of a balanced diet and provided practical tips for meal planning and preparation. For the first time in a long while, Lisa felt empowered.

The real magic began when Lisa ventured into the chapters filled with recipes. Each dish was thoughtfully crafted, taking into account the dietary restrictions while ensuring flavor and satisfaction were not compromised. Breakfast options like Spinach and Mushroom Omelette and Blueberry Almond Overnight Oats rekindled her love for morning meals. Lunches were no longer a struggle, with recipes like Grilled Chicken Salad with Lemon Vinaigrette and Baked Cod with Steamed Broccoli offering delicious and nutritious choices.

Dinner, once a daunting task, became a highlight of her day. Lisa delighted in making Herb-Crusted Salmon with Asparagus and Stuffed Bell Peppers with Ground Turkey. The recipes were easy to follow, with clear instructions and accessible ingredients. The cookbook even included snacks, sides, desserts, and beverages, ensuring every craving was met without compromising her health.

What truly set the "Diabetic Renal Diet Cookbook for Beginners 2024" apart was its comprehensive approach. Beyond the recipes, it provided sample meal plans, shopping lists, and lifestyle tips for managing diabetes and kidney disease. Lisa learned how to stay active, manage stress, and even enjoy dining out without worry. The appendices, filled with nutritional information and a glossary of terms, became her go-to resources.

As Lisa's confidence grew, so did her health. She felt more energetic, her blood sugar levels stabilized, and her kidney function improved. Mark noticed the change too—Lisa was smiling more, her laughter filling their home once again. Cooking, once a source of frustration, became a shared joy as they explored new recipes together.

Lisa's story spread through their community, inspiring others facing similar challenges. She often found herself recommending the cookbook to friends and family, sharing her journey of transformation. The "Diabetic Renal Diet Cookbook for Beginners 2024" had not just provided recipes; it had given Lisa and her loved ones a new lease on life.

In the end, Lisa realized that the cookbook was more than just a collection of recipes—it was a guide to reclaiming health and happiness. It offered hope, knowledge, and the tools needed to navigate the complexities of a diabetic renal diet. For anyone facing the dual challenges of diabetes and kidney disease, this book was a beacon of light, guiding them towards a healthier, more fulfilling life.

And so, Lisa's kitchen was once again filled with the aromas of delicious meals, but now, each dish was a testament to resilience, love, and the power of the right guide to make all the difference.

Understanding Diabetes and Kidney Disease

Diabetes and kidney disease are closely linked conditions that require careful management, particularly when it comes to diet. Diabetes, a chronic condition characterized by high blood sugar levels, can damage the kidneys over time. The kidneys play a crucial role in filtering waste and excess fluids from the blood. When diabetes is not well-controlled, the high blood sugar levels can harm these filtering units, leading to a condition known as diabetic nephropathy. This condition is a leading cause of chronic kidney disease (CKD) and can progress to kidney failure if not properly managed.

People with diabetes and kidney disease need to follow a specific diet to help manage their conditions and prevent further damage. This diet is often referred to as a diabetic renal diet. It focuses on controlling blood sugar levels, reducing the workload on the kidneys, and maintaining overall health. Key components of this diet include limiting the intake of certain nutrients such as sodium, potassium, and phosphorus, which can be harmful in large amounts for people with compromised kidney function.

Managing diabetes and kidney disease through diet involves balancing the intake of carbohydrates, proteins, and fats. Carbohydrates have the most significant impact on blood sugar levels, so it is essential to choose complex carbohydrates that release sugar slowly into the bloodstream. Whole grains, vegetables, and legumes are excellent sources of these complex carbs. Protein intake must also be carefully monitored, as the kidneys need to work harder to process proteins. Lean protein sources like fish, chicken, and plant-based proteins are preferable over red meats and processed foods.

Sodium control is another critical aspect of the diabetic renal diet. Excessive sodium can lead to high blood pressure, which further damages the kidneys. Therefore, it is important to avoid processed foods, canned soups, and salty snacks. Instead, opt for fresh, whole foods and season meals with herbs and spices rather than salt. Potassium and phosphorus are also minerals that need to be controlled in this diet. High levels of these minerals can accumulate in the blood when the kidneys are not functioning correctly, leading to serious health issues.

Hydration is important, but it needs to be balanced. While staying hydrated helps the kidneys function properly, fluid intake might need to be restricted depending on the stage of kidney disease. Drinking plenty of water is usually recommended, but individuals with advanced kidney disease might need to limit their fluid intake to avoid overloading the kidneys. Consulting with a healthcare provider or a dietitian is crucial to determine the right amount of fluid intake.

A diabetic renal diet is not just about restriction; it's also about making healthier food choices and enjoying a variety of foods that support overall well-being. Fresh fruits and vegetables, low-fat dairy products, and healthy fats from sources like olive oil, avocados, and nuts can be included in moderation. Meal planning and preparation become vital skills in managing diabetes and kidney disease. Learning to read nutrition labels, cook at home, and plan meals ahead can make a significant difference in maintaining health and preventing complications.

Living with diabetes and kidney disease requires a comprehensive approach to diet and lifestyle. It involves understanding the interplay between the two conditions and how diet can influence health outcomes. By following a carefully designed diabetic renal diet, individuals can take proactive steps to manage their conditions, improve their quality of life, and prevent further health complications. The "Diabetic Renal Diet Cookbook for Beginners 2024" is an invaluable resource that offers guidance, delicious recipes, and practical tips to help individuals navigate this challenging journey.

Benefits of a Diabetic Renal Diet

A diabetic renal diet is essential for managing the dual challenges of diabetes and kidney disease, as it helps to balance blood sugar levels while protecting kidney function. This diet, carefully crafted with the principles laid out in the Diabetic Renal Diet Cookbook for Beginners 2024, offers numerous benefits that go beyond merely addressing health concerns. It fosters a holistic approach to well-being that transforms lives by making dietary management both accessible and enjoyable.

One of the key benefits of this diet is the stabilization of blood sugar levels. By focusing on low-glycemic index foods and balanced meals, it helps prevent the spikes and crashes that can occur with diabetes. The recipes in the cookbook are designed to provide a steady release of energy, which is crucial for maintaining consistent blood glucose levels. This stability not only reduces the risk of complications associated with diabetes but also enhances overall energy levels and mood.

Protecting kidney function is another critical advantage of the diabetic renal diet. The diet emphasizes foods that are low in sodium, potassium, and phosphorus, which are essential for kidney health. Overloading the kidneys with these minerals can lead to further damage, but the cookbook offers a variety of recipes that are both delicious and kidney-friendly. By reducing the intake of harmful substances, the diet helps to slow the progression of kidney disease and maintain optimal renal function.

Weight management is often a challenging aspect of living with diabetes and kidney disease. The diabetic renal diet aids in achieving and maintaining a healthy weight by promoting nutrient-dense, low-calorie foods that are satisfying and flavorful. The meal plans and recipes in the cookbook encourage portion control and balanced nutrition, making it easier to avoid overeating and manage weight effectively. This approach not only supports kidney health but also reduces the risk of other obesity-related conditions.

The cookbook also highlights the importance of heart health, which is particularly vital for individuals with diabetes and kidney disease. The diet includes heart-healthy fats, lean proteins, and high-fiber foods that help reduce cholesterol levels and improve cardiovascular health. The inclusion of these nutrient-rich foods helps to mitigate the increased risk of heart disease, which is a common complication in individuals managing both diabetes and kidney issues.

Adopting a diabetic renal diet can significantly improve digestion and reduce gastrointestinal discomfort. The focus on whole foods, fiber, and proper hydration supports healthy digestion and prevents issues such as constipation and bloating. The cookbook provides recipes that are easy on the digestive system, ensuring that meals are not only nutritious but also comfortable to consume, enhancing the overall quality of life.

Emotional well-being is another often-overlooked benefit of the diabetic renal diet. The stress of managing two chronic conditions can take a toll on mental health, but having a clear, structured dietary plan can alleviate some of this burden. The Diabetic Renal Diet Cookbook for Beginners 2024 offers guidance and inspiration, helping individuals feel more in control of their health. This sense of empowerment and the joy of discovering tasty, healthful meals can boost self-esteem and improve mental outlook.

Ultimately, the diabetic renal diet fosters a sustainable, long-term approach to health. It encourages lifestyle changes that are manageable and realistic, promoting lasting habits that support both diabetes and kidney health. The comprehensive nature of the cookbook, with its practical tips, varied recipes, and meal plans, makes it an invaluable resource for anyone looking to improve their health. By embracing this diet, individuals can look forward to a future of better health, increased vitality, and enhanced quality of life.

Essential Nutrients for Kidney Health

Maintaining kidney health is crucial for individuals managing both diabetes and kidney disease. One of the most vital aspects of this is understanding the essential nutrients that support kidney function while also keeping blood sugar levels in check. A balanced diet tailored to these needs can significantly impact overall health and well-being. It's important to focus on incorporating foods that are low in phosphorus, potassium, and sodium while being rich in vitamins and minerals that promote kidney health and help manage diabetes.

Protein intake should be carefully monitored. While protein is essential for the body's repair and maintenance, too much can put a strain on the kidneys. Lean proteins such as fish, chicken, and plant-based options like beans and lentils are preferable. These sources provide the necessary nutrients without the excess phosphorus and potassium found in many animal products. The key is to consume these proteins in moderation, ensuring that the diet supports kidney function without overloading the organs.

Carbohydrates are another critical component, particularly in managing diabetes. Complex carbohydrates, such as whole grains, vegetables, and fruits, should be prioritized over simple sugars and processed foods. These complex carbs provide a slow and steady release of glucose, helping to maintain stable blood sugar levels. Additionally, they are often rich in fiber, which is beneficial for digestive health and can help in controlling blood sugar levels. However, portion control is essential to prevent spikes in blood sugar.

Fats are necessary for overall health, but the type and quantity are crucial. Unsaturated fats, found in olive oil, avocados, and nuts, are beneficial and can help reduce inflammation, which is particularly important for individuals with kidney disease. These healthy fats also support heart health, which is often a concern for diabetic patients. Saturated fats and trans fats, commonly found in fried foods and baked goods, should be limited as they can contribute to cardiovascular disease and exacerbate kidney issues.

Micronutrients play a significant role in kidney health. Vitamin D is crucial as it helps regulate calcium and phosphorus levels in the blood, which is essential for kidney function. Foods like fortified cereals and fatty fish can be good sources. However, since people with kidney disease often need to limit phosphorus intake, it's essential to balance these sources appropriately. Additionally, iron is important for preventing anemia, a common issue in kidney disease patients, and can be found in lean meats, beans, and fortified grains.

Hydration is another key factor in maintaining kidney health. Drinking sufficient water helps the kidneys remove waste and toxins from the blood. However, fluid intake needs to be managed carefully for those with kidney disease to prevent overloading the kidneys. It's advisable to spread water intake throughout the day and avoid high-sodium foods that can lead to water retention and high blood pressure, further stressing the kidneys.

Sodium intake should be kept low to manage both kidney health and blood pressure. High sodium levels can lead to fluid retention and increased blood pressure, which can damage the kidneys over time. Cooking at home with fresh ingredients and avoiding processed and packaged foods can significantly reduce sodium intake. Using herbs and spices instead of salt can enhance the flavor of food without the negative impact on health.

Balancing these essential nutrients is a delicate process, but it's vital for those managing diabetes and kidney disease. The recipes and meal plans in the Diabetic Renal Diet Cookbook for Beginners 2024 are designed with this balance in mind, ensuring that each meal supports kidney health while helping to maintain stable blood sugar levels. By focusing on the right types of proteins, carbohydrates, fats, and micronutrients, and by managing fluid and sodium intake, individuals can enjoy delicious meals that contribute to their overall health and well-being.

Tips for Meal Planning and Preparation

When embarking on a journey with the diabetic renal diet, meal planning and preparation become essential tools in maintaining health and managing both diabetes and kidney disease. The first step is to understand the specific dietary requirements associated with these conditions. It involves limiting sodium, potassium, and phosphorus intake while ensuring that meals are balanced with the right amounts of protein, carbohydrates, and fats. This knowledge serves as the foundation for effective meal planning, helping to create menus that support overall health and well-being.

A key aspect of successful meal planning is organization. Start by mapping out your meals for the week, taking into consideration your daily nutritional needs and personal preferences. Planning ahead allows you to create a grocery list that includes all the necessary ingredients, reducing the temptation to make unhealthy food choices. It also helps to avoid last-minute stress, ensuring that you always have the right foods on hand. Batch cooking and preparing ingredients in advance can save time during the week, making it easier to stick to your diet plan.

Incorporating a variety of fresh, whole foods is crucial. Focus on including a range of fruits, vegetables, whole grains, and lean proteins in your meals. For instance, opting for low-potassium vegetables like bell peppers, carrots, and green beans can help manage kidney health. Similarly, choosing whole grains such as quinoa or brown rice over refined grains can provide essential nutrients without spiking blood sugar levels. Variety not only ensures a broader spectrum of nutrients but also keeps meals interesting and enjoyable.

Cooking methods play a significant role in maintaining the nutritional value of your food. Opt for baking, grilling, steaming, or sautéing instead of frying to reduce unhealthy fats. Using herbs and spices to season your meals can enhance flavor without adding excess sodium. Fresh herbs like basil, cilantro, and parsley, along with spices such as turmeric, ginger, and cumin, can make a big difference. Experimenting with different seasonings can make your meals more enjoyable and satisfying, helping you adhere to your diet more easily.

Portion control is another important aspect of managing both diabetes and kidney disease. Eating smaller, more frequent meals can help keep blood sugar levels stable and prevent overeating. Measuring your portions and being mindful of serving sizes can ensure that you're not consuming too much of any one nutrient. This approach also helps in maintaining a healthy weight, which is beneficial for overall health management. Keeping a food diary can be a useful tool in tracking what you eat and making adjustments as needed.

Staying hydrated is essential, but it's important to monitor fluid intake when dealing with kidney disease. Drinking the right amount of water and choosing low-potassium beverages can help manage your condition. Infused waters with slices of cucumber, lemon, or berries can be a refreshing alternative to sugary drinks. Avoiding sodas and high-sugar beverages is crucial, as they can contribute to both blood sugar spikes and kidney damage. Staying hydrated with the right fluids supports your overall health and complements your meal plan.

Support and resources can make a significant difference in maintaining a diabetic renal diet. Engaging with a dietitian or nutritionist can provide personalized guidance tailored to your specific health needs. Joining support groups or online communities can offer encouragement and share practical tips from others facing similar challenges. Utilizing cookbooks like the "Diabetic Renal Diet Cookbook for Beginners 2024" can provide a wealth of recipes and ideas to keep your meals exciting and nutritious. With the right tools and support, meal planning and preparation become manageable, empowering you to take control of your health and enjoy delicious, kidney-friendly meals.

How to Use This Cookbook

The "Diabetic Renal Diet Cookbook for Beginners 2024" is designed to be your companion in navigating the complexities of managing both diabetes and kidney disease through diet. To make the most of this cookbook, start by familiarizing yourself with the foundational principles outlined in the initial chapters. These sections provide essential information about the specific dietary needs associated with both conditions, ensuring you understand the importance of balancing nutrients, controlling portion sizes, and selecting the right ingredients.

As you delve into the recipes, you will find each one crafted with careful consideration of the dietary restrictions necessary for managing diabetes and kidney health. The ingredient lists and step-by-step instructions are straightforward and easy to follow, allowing you to prepare meals with confidence. Pay close attention to the portion sizes recommended in each recipe, as portion control is crucial in maintaining stable blood sugar levels and managing kidney function effectively.

Meal planning is an integral part of successfully following a diabetic renal diet. Use the cookbook to create weekly meal plans that incorporate a variety of recipes from each section—breakfast, lunch, dinner, snacks, and desserts. This variety not only keeps your meals interesting and enjoyable but also ensures a balanced intake of essential nutrients.

Take advantage of the sample meal plans provided in the cookbook to get started, and gradually adapt them to suit your personal preferences and lifestyle.

Shopping for ingredients can be a challenge, but the cookbook includes practical tips and comprehensive shopping lists to simplify this process. Focus on fresh, whole foods, and try to avoid processed items that may contain hidden sugars, sodium, or phosphorus. The ingredient substitutions suggested in the cookbook can also help you adapt recipes to what is available locally or to accommodate personal tastes and dietary restrictions.

As you prepare and enjoy the meals, pay attention to how your body responds to different foods. Everyone's health journey is unique, and you may find that certain ingredients or meal combinations work better for you. Keep a food diary to track your meals, blood sugar levels, and kidney function, which can help you identify patterns and make informed adjustments to your diet. The cookbook encourages this mindful eating approach, empowering you to take control of your health.

Beyond the recipes, the cookbook offers valuable lifestyle tips to support your overall well-being. Staying active, managing stress, and maintaining a positive mindset are all critical components of managing diabetes and kidney disease. The book provides practical advice on incorporating gentle exercises into your daily routine, techniques for reducing stress, and tips for maintaining motivation and a positive outlook on your health journey.

Finally, remember that this cookbook is more than just a collection of recipes; it is a resource designed to support you every step of the way. Whether you are new to cooking or an experienced home chef, the "Diabetic Renal Diet Cookbook for Beginners 2024" offers the guidance, inspiration, and tools needed to create delicious, healthy meals that nourish your body and enhance your quality of life. Embrace this journey with an open heart and a willingness to explore new flavors and techniques, knowing that each meal you prepare brings you closer to achieving your health goals.

Chapter 1: Breakfast Delights

Spinach and Mushroom Omelette

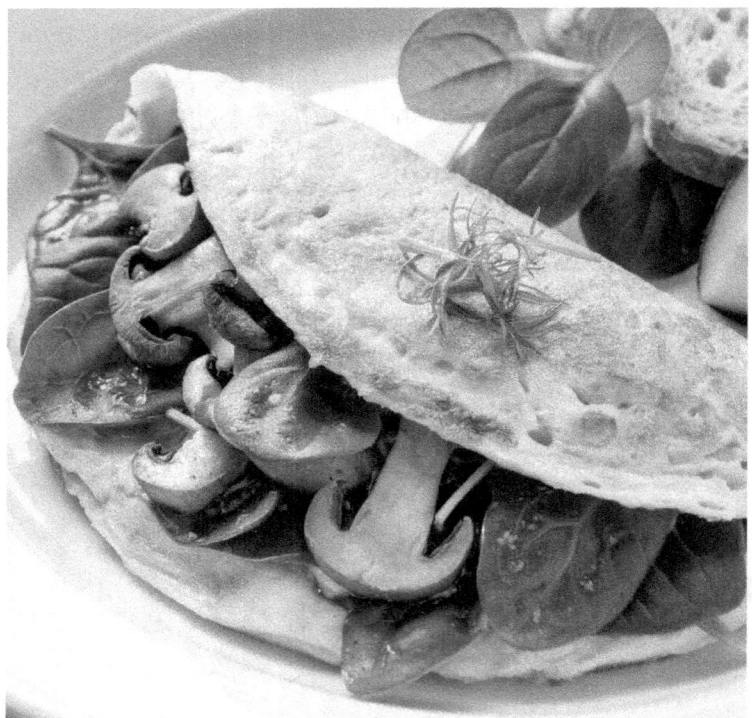

Ingredients:

- 1 cup fresh spinach, chopped
- 1/2 cup mushrooms, sliced
- 2 large eggs or egg substitute equivalent
- 1/4 cup low-fat milk or milk substitute

- 1/4 teaspoon black pepper
- 1/4 teaspoon onion powder
- 1/4 teaspoon garlic powder
- 1 teaspoon olive oil

Instructions:

1. Heat the olive oil in a non-stick skillet over medium heat.
2. Add the mushrooms and cook for 3-4 minutes until they start to soften.
3. Add the spinach and cook for another 2 minutes until wilted. Remove the vegetables from the skillet and set aside.
4. In a bowl, whisk the eggs, milk, black pepper, onion powder, and garlic powder together until well combined.
5. Pour the egg mixture into the skillet and cook without stirring until the eggs start to set.
6. Add the spinach and mushrooms evenly over one half of the omelette.
7. Carefully fold the other half of the omelette over the vegetables.
8. Continue cooking for another 1-2 minutes until the omelette is fully set.
9. Slide the omelette onto a plate and serve immediately.

Nutritional Information:

- Calories: 210
- Protein: 14g
- Carbohydrates: 5g
- Dietary Fiber: 2g

- Sugars: 2g
- Fat: 14g
- Sodium: 200mg
- Potassium: 350mg

Serving Size:
1 omelette

Cooking Time:
10 minutes

Blueberry Almond Overnight Oats

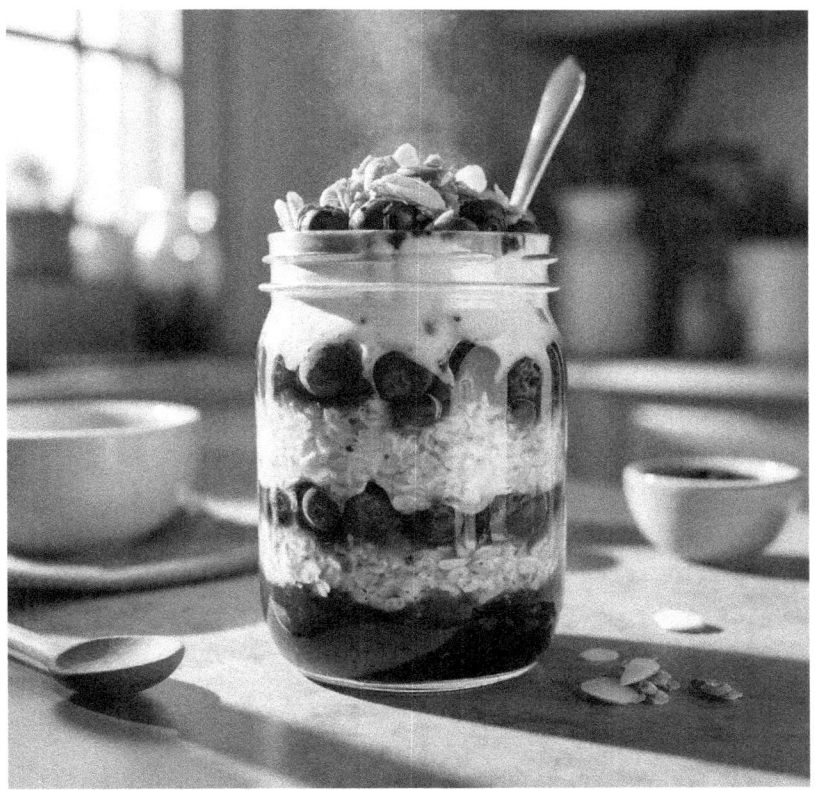

For the Blueberry Almond Overnight Oats, gather the following ingredients:

- 1/2 cup old-fashioned oats
- 1/2 cup unsweetened almond milk
- 1/4 cup fresh or frozen blueberries
- 1 tablespoon almond butter

- 1 teaspoon chia seeds
- 1/2 teaspoon vanilla extract
- A pinch of ground cinnamon
- A few almond slices for topping (optional)

Instructions:

1. In a mason jar or a small bowl, combine the oats, almond milk, almond butter, chia seeds, vanilla extract, and ground cinnamon. Stir well to ensure all ingredients are mixed thoroughly.
2. Add the blueberries on top of the mixture. You can gently stir them in or leave them on top.
3. Cover the jar or bowl with a lid or plastic wrap and refrigerate overnight, or for at least 4 hours.
4. In the morning, give the oats a good stir. If the mixture is too thick, add a splash of almond milk to reach your desired consistency.
5. Top with almond slices if desired, and enjoy your nutritious breakfast.

Nutritional Information (per serving):

- Calories: 250
- Protein: 7 grams
- Carbohydrates: 36 grams
- Dietary Fiber: 8 grams
- Sugars: 8 grams
- Fat: 9 grams
- Sodium: 100 mg

- Potassium: 150 mg

Serving Size: 1 jar or bowl (recipe makes 1 serving)

Cooking Time: 10 minutes preparation, plus overnight refrigeration

Greek Yogurt with Fresh Berries and Chia Seeds

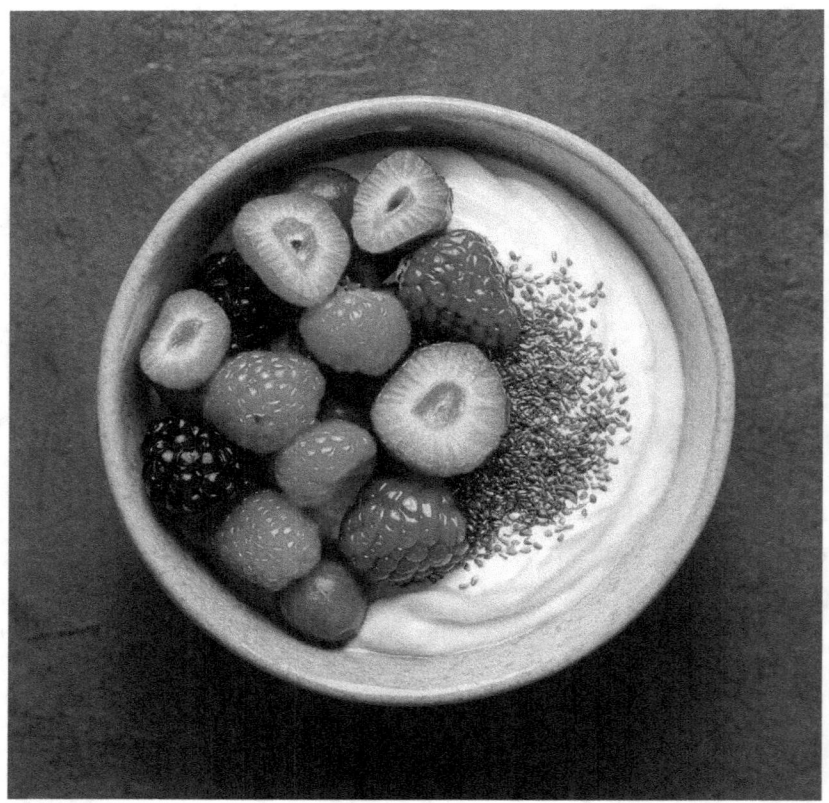

Ingredient:

- 1 cup plain Greek yogurt
- 1/2 cup fresh mixed berries (such as strawberries, blueberries, and raspberries)
- 1 tablespoon chia seeds

- 1 teaspoon honey (optional)
- 1/4 teaspoon vanilla extract (optional)

Instructions:

1. In a bowl, mix the plain Greek yogurt with the vanilla extract if using.
2. Layer the fresh mixed berries on top of the yogurt.
3. Sprinkle the chia seeds over the berries.
4. Drizzle with honey if desired.
5. Stir gently to combine all ingredients or serve layered as is.

Nutritional Information (per serving):

- Calories: 180
- Protein: 15g
- Carbohydrates: 20g
- Dietary Fiber: 5g
- Sugars: 12g (including natural sugars from berries)
- Fat: 6g
- Sodium: 60mg
- Potassium: 220mg
- Phosphorus: 200mg

Serving Size: 1 bowl

Cooking Time: 5 minutes

Quinoa Breakfast Bowl with Apples and Cinnamon

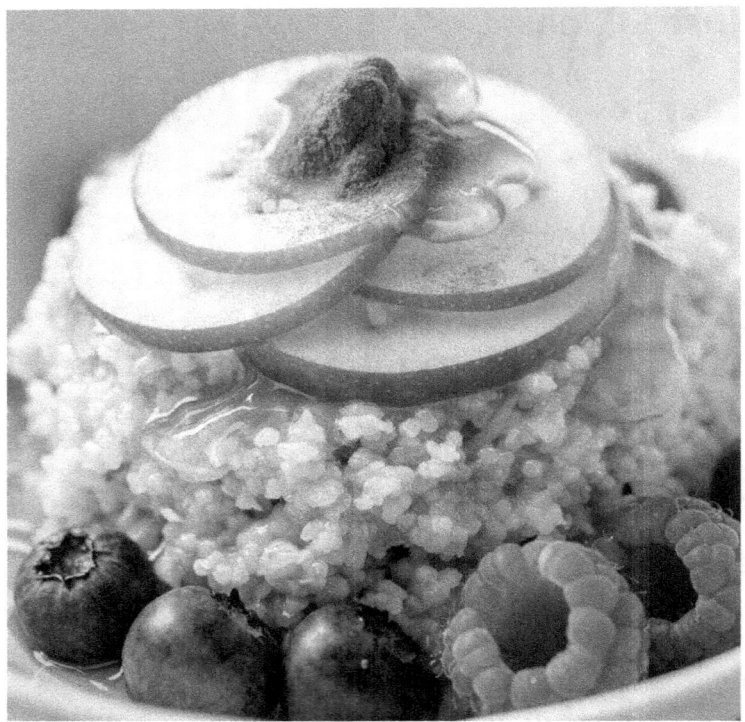

Ingredients:

- 1 cup quinoa, rinsed
- 2 cups water
- 1 medium apple, chopped
- 1 teaspoon ground cinnamon
- 1 tablespoon chia seeds
- 1/4 cup unsweetened almond milk

- 1 tablespoon maple syrup (optional)
- 1/4 cup chopped walnuts (optional)

Instructions:

1. In a medium saucepan, combine quinoa and water. Bring to a boil, then reduce heat to low, cover, and simmer for 15 minutes or until quinoa is tender and water is absorbed.
2. While the quinoa is cooking, chop the apple and set it aside.
3. Once the quinoa is cooked, remove it from the heat and let it sit, covered, for 5 minutes.
4. Fluff the quinoa with a fork and stir in the chopped apple, ground cinnamon, and chia seeds.
5. Divide the quinoa mixture into bowls and drizzle with unsweetened almond milk.
6. If desired, add a tablespoon of maple syrup for extra sweetness and sprinkle with chopped walnuts.

Nutritional Information (per serving):

- Calories: 250
- Protein: 7g
- Carbohydrates: 42g
- Dietary Fiber: 6g
- Sugars: 9g
- Fat: 6g
- Sodium: 10mg
- Potassium: 220mg
- Phosphorus: 150mg

Serving Size:
- Serves 2

Cooking Time:
- Total: 25 minutes

Scrambled Tofu with Vegetables

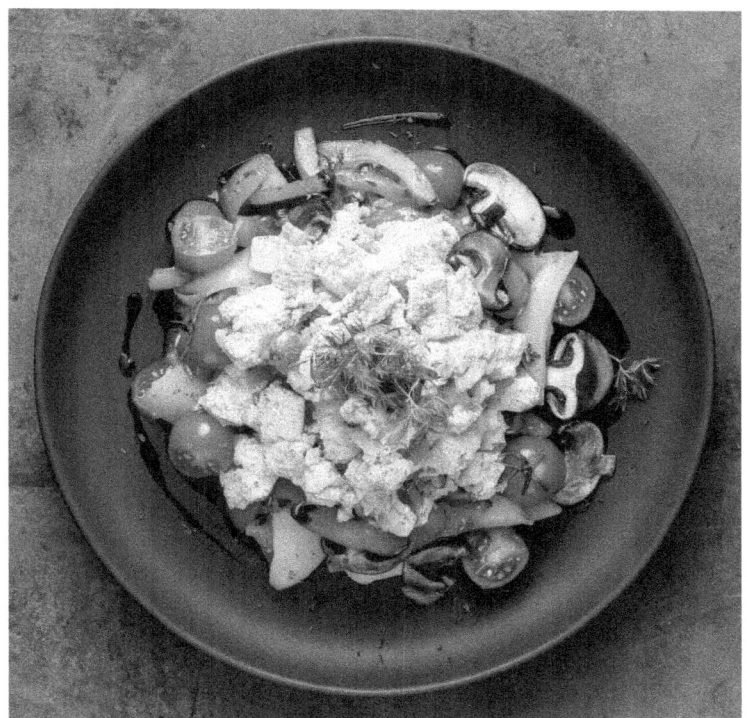

Ingredients:
- 1 block of firm tofu, drained and crumbled
- 1 tablespoon olive oil
- 1/2 cup diced bell peppers (any color)
- 1/2 cup diced tomatoes
- 1/4 cup chopped spinach
- 1/4 cup diced onions
- 1 clove garlic, minced

- 1/2 teaspoon turmeric
- Salt and pepper to taste
- Fresh parsley for garnish

Instructions:

1. Heat the olive oil in a large non-stick skillet over medium heat.
2. Add the diced onions and garlic, sautéing until they become translucent.
3. Stir in the bell peppers and tomatoes, cooking until they begin to soften.
4. Add the crumbled tofu to the skillet, mixing well with the vegetables.
5. Sprinkle the turmeric over the tofu mixture, stirring to ensure even coloring.
6. Add the chopped spinach, allowing it to wilt into the scramble.
7. Season with salt and pepper to taste, cooking for an additional 3-4 minutes until everything is heated through.
8. Garnish with fresh parsley before serving.

Nutritional Information (per serving):

- Calories: 180
- Protein: 14g
- Carbohydrates: 8g
- Fiber: 3g
- Fat: 11g
- Sodium: 150mg

- Potassium: 300mg

Serving Size:
- Serves 2

Cooking Time:
- Total: 20 minutes

Whole Grain Avocado Toast

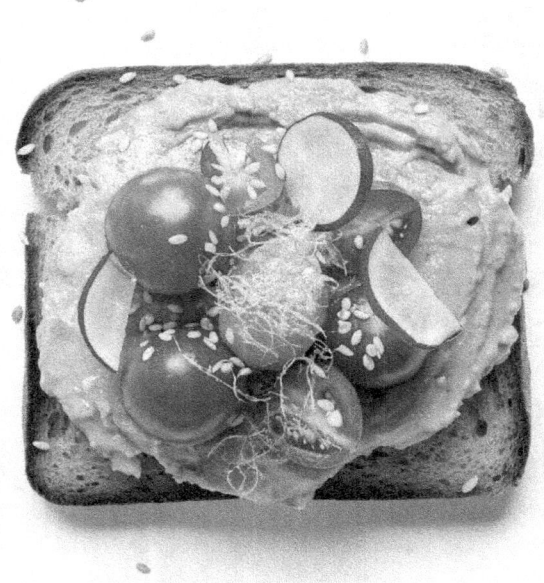

Ingredient:

- 1 slice of whole grain bread
- 1/2 ripe avocado
- A pinch of salt
- A squeeze of fresh lemon juice
- Optional: cherry tomatoes, fresh herbs, or a sprinkle of red pepper flakes for garnish

Instructions:

1. Toast the slice of whole grain bread until golden brown.
2. While the bread is toasting, cut the avocado in half, remove the pit, and scoop the flesh into a bowl.
3. Mash the avocado with a fork until smooth. Add a pinch of salt and a squeeze of fresh lemon juice, mixing well.
4. Spread the mashed avocado evenly over the toasted bread.
5. If desired, top with cherry tomatoes, fresh herbs, or a sprinkle of red pepper flakes for extra flavor.

Nutritional Information:

- Calories: 180
- Protein: 4g
- Carbohydrates: 20g
- Fiber: 7g
- Total Fat: 11g
- Saturated Fat: 1.5g
- Sodium: 150mg
- Potassium: 500mg
- Phosphorus: 110mg

Serving Size:

- 1 slice

Cooking Time:

- 5 minutes

Berry and Spinach Smoothie

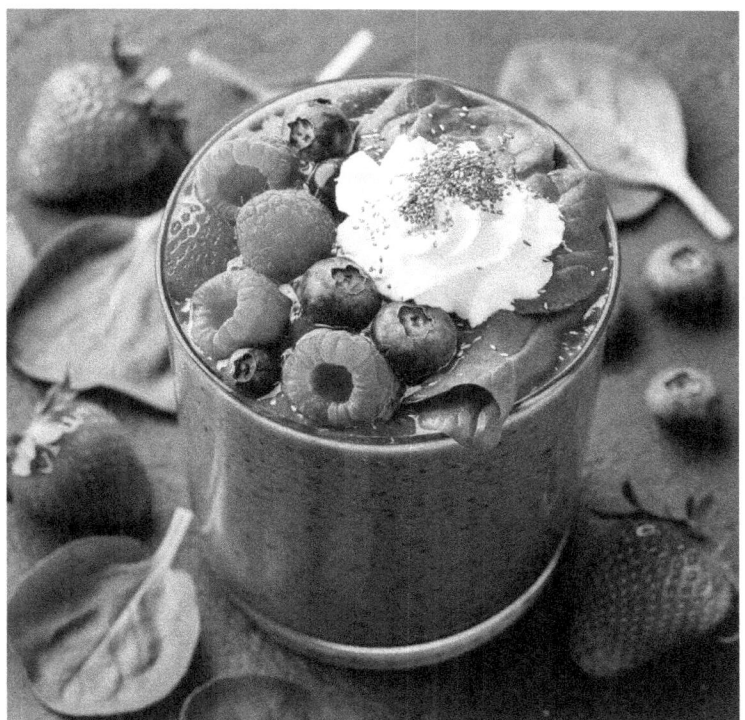

Ingredient:
- 1 cup fresh spinach leaves
- 1/2 cup frozen mixed berries (such as strawberries, blueberries, and raspberries)
- 1/2 banana
- 1/2 cup unsweetened almond milk
- 1/4 cup plain Greek yogurt
- 1 tablespoon chia seeds

- 1 teaspoon honey (optional)

Instructions:

1. Rinse the spinach leaves thoroughly and pat them dry.
2. Place the spinach, frozen berries, banana, almond milk, Greek yogurt, and chia seeds in a blender.
3. Blend on high speed until the mixture is smooth and creamy.
4. Taste the smoothie and add honey if you prefer a sweeter taste.
5. Pour the smoothie into a glass and serve immediately.

Nutritional Information (per serving):

- Calories: 150
- Protein: 7g
- Carbohydrates: 28g
- Dietary Fiber: 6g
- Sugars: 16g
- Fat: 3g
- Sodium: 55mg
- Potassium: 350mg
- Phosphorus: 130mg

Serving Size: 1 glass (approximately 12 ounces)

Cooking Time: 5 minutes

Cottage Cheese with Pineapple

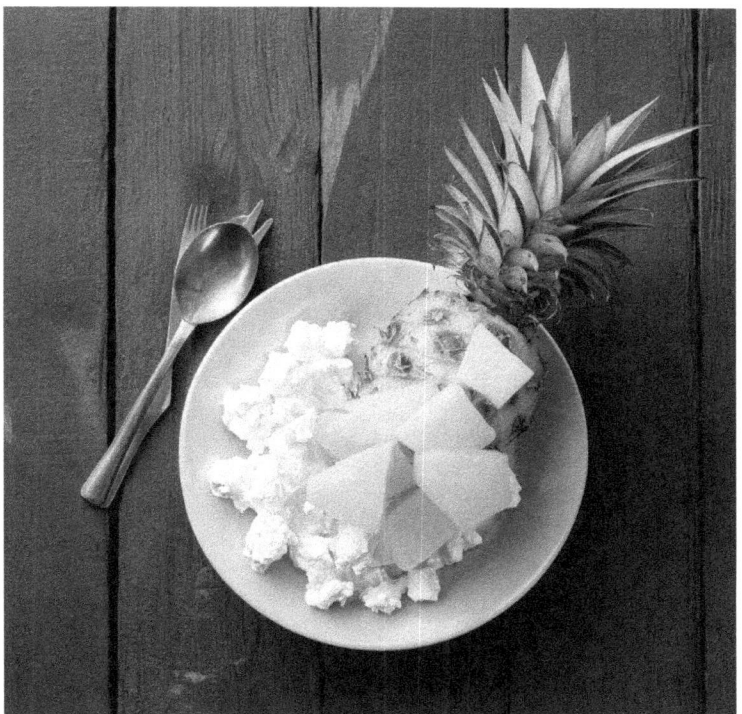

Ingredients:

- 1 cup low-fat cottage cheese
- 1/2 cup fresh pineapple chunks
- 1 tablespoon chopped fresh mint (optional)
- 1 teaspoon honey (optional)

Instructions:
1. Place the cottage cheese in a serving bowl.

2. Top with fresh pineapple chunks.
3. If desired, drizzle with honey and sprinkle with chopped fresh mint.
4. Serve immediately and enjoy!

Nutritional Information:

- Calories: 120
- Protein: 14g
- Carbohydrates: 12g
- Fiber: 1g
- Sugars: 10g
- Fat: 2g
- Sodium: 400mg
- Potassium: 180mg
- Phosphorus: 170mg

Serving Size:

- 1 serving (approximately 1 1/2 cups)

Cooking Time:

- 5 minutes

Low-Sodium Turkey and Egg White Breakfast Wrap

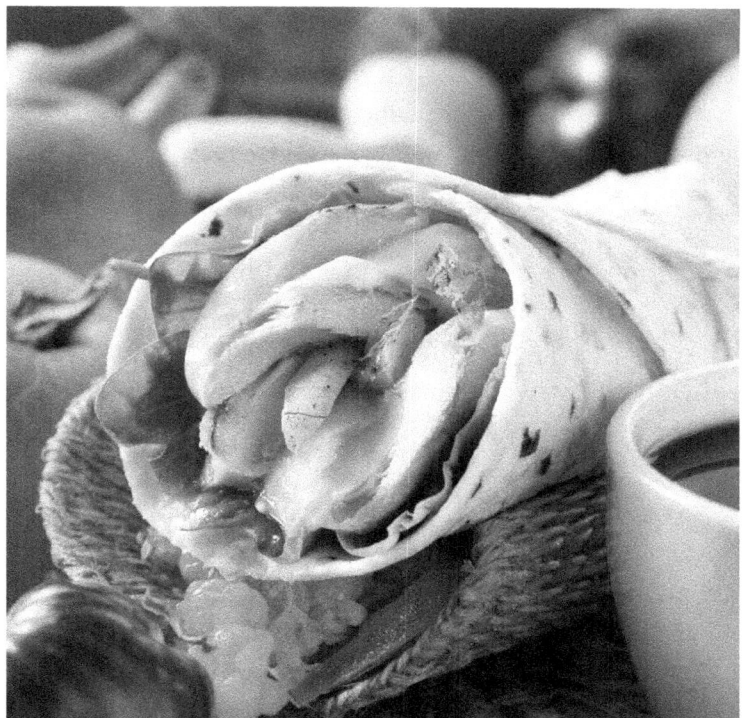

Ingredients:

- 4 egg whites
- 2 slices of low-sodium turkey breast
- 1/4 cup chopped spinach
- 1/4 cup diced tomatoes
- 1/4 cup shredded low-fat cheese (optional)
- 1 whole-wheat tortilla

- 1 tablespoon olive oil
- Salt and pepper to taste

Instructions:

1. Heat the olive oil in a non-stick skillet over medium heat.
2. Add the chopped spinach and diced tomatoes to the skillet and sauté for 2-3 minutes until the spinach is wilted.
3. In a small bowl, whisk the egg whites with a pinch of salt and pepper.
4. Pour the egg whites into the skillet with the vegetables and cook, stirring frequently, until the egg whites are fully cooked.
5. Lay the whole-wheat tortilla flat on a clean surface. Place the cooked egg whites and vegetables in the center of the tortilla.
6. Layer the low-sodium turkey breast slices on top of the egg mixture. Add the shredded low-fat cheese if desired.
7. Fold the sides of the tortilla over the filling and then roll it up tightly to form a wrap.
8. Place the wrap back in the skillet and cook for an additional 1-2 minutes on each side until the tortilla is lightly browned and crispy.

Nutritional Information:

- Calories: 250
- Protein: 20g
- Carbohydrates: 20g
- Dietary Fiber: 5g

- Sugars: 2g
- Fat: 10g
- Saturated Fat: 2g
- Sodium: 300mg
- Potassium: 350mg
- Phosphorus: 200mg

Serving Size:
- 1 wrap

Cooking Time:
- 15 minutes

Spiced Apple and Oat Muffins

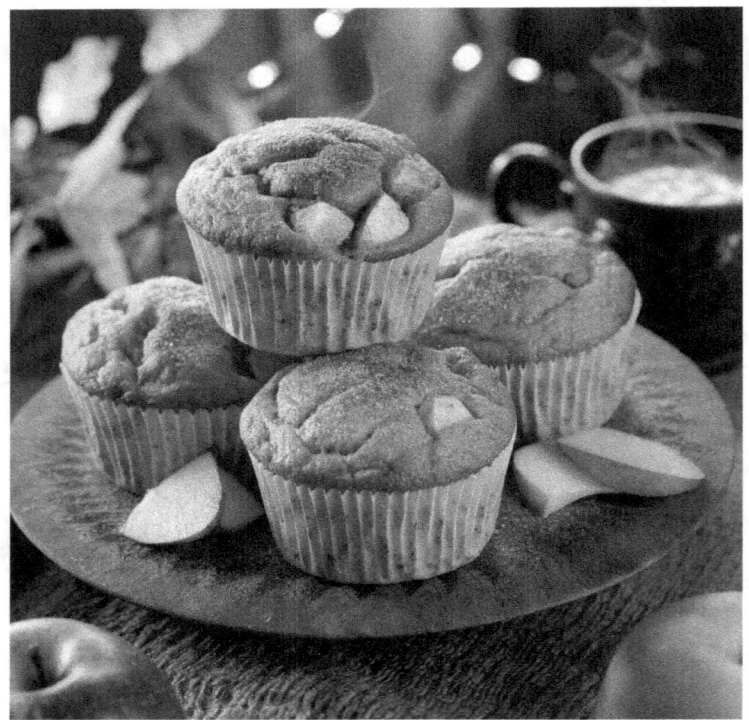

Ingredients

- 1 cup rolled oats
- 1 cup whole wheat flour
- 1 teaspoon baking powder
- 1/2 teaspoon baking soda
- 1/2 teaspoon ground cinnamon
- 1/4 teaspoon ground nutmeg
- 1/4 teaspoon salt

- 1/2 cup unsweetened applesauce
- 1/2 cup low-fat milk or a plant-based alternative
- 1/4 cup honey or a sugar substitute suitable for baking
- 1 large egg
- 1 teaspoon vanilla extract
- 1 medium apple, peeled, cored, and finely chopped

Instructions

1. Preheat your oven to 375°F (190°C) and line a muffin tin with paper liners or lightly grease it.
2. In a large bowl, combine the rolled oats, whole wheat flour, baking powder, baking soda, cinnamon, nutmeg, and salt.
3. In a separate bowl, whisk together the applesauce, milk, honey, egg, and vanilla extract until well combined.
4. Pour the wet ingredients into the dry ingredients and stir until just combined.
5. Gently fold in the chopped apple.
6. Divide the batter evenly among the prepared muffin cups, filling each about two-thirds full.

Nutritional Information

- Calories: 140 per muffin
- Protein: 3 grams
- Carbohydrates: 26 grams
- Dietary Fiber: 3 grams
- Sugars: 10 grams
- Fat: 3 grams
- Sodium: 120 milligrams

- Potassium: 85 milligrams

Serving Size
- 1 muffin

Cooking Time
- Total: 30 minutes (Prep: 10 minutes, Cook: 20 minutes)

Chapter 2: Lunch Solutions

Grilled Chicken Salad with Lemon Vinaigrette

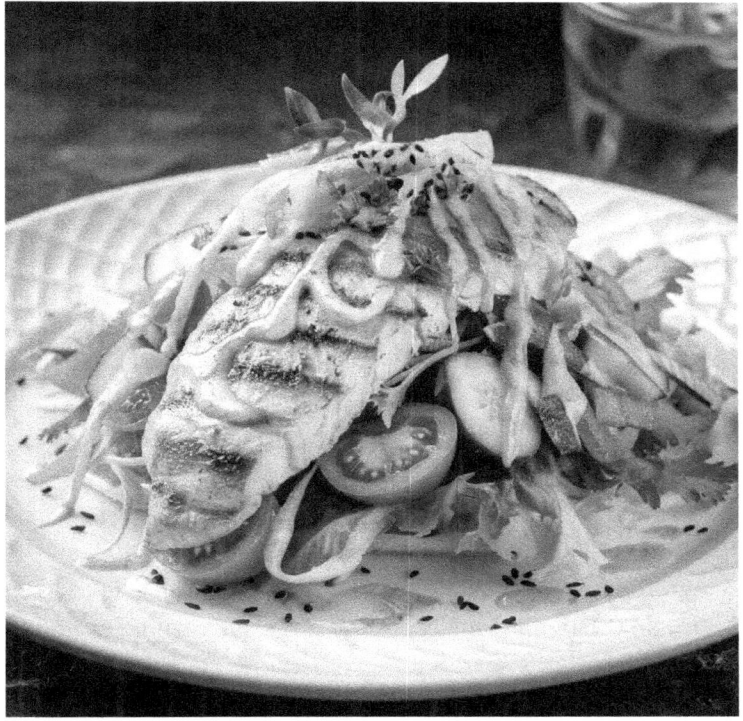

Ingredient:

- 1 boneless, skinless chicken breast
- 4 cups mixed greens (e.g., spinach, arugula, romaine)
- 1/2 cup cherry tomatoes, halved

- 1/4 cup cucumber, sliced
- 1/4 cup red bell pepper, sliced
- 1/4 cup red onion, thinly sliced
- 1 tablespoon olive oil
- 1 tablespoon lemon juice
- 1 teaspoon Dijon mustard
- 1 clove garlic, minced
- Salt and pepper to taste

Instructions:

1. Preheat the grill to medium-high heat.
2. Season the chicken breast with salt and pepper.
3. Grill the chicken for 5-7 minutes on each side, or until fully cooked and the internal temperature reaches 165°F. Let it rest for a few minutes before slicing.
4. In a small bowl, whisk together the olive oil, lemon juice, Dijon mustard, minced garlic, and a pinch of salt and pepper to make the vinaigrette.
5. In a large bowl, combine the mixed greens, cherry tomatoes, cucumber, red bell pepper, and red onion.
6. Add the grilled chicken slices on top of the salad.
7. Drizzle the lemon vinaigrette over the salad and toss gently to combine.
8. Serve immediately.

Nutritional Information:

- Calories: 320
- Protein: 30g

- Carbohydrates: 12g
- Dietary Fiber: 4g
- Sugars: 5g
- Fat: 18g
- Saturated Fat: 3g
- Sodium: 210mg
- Potassium: 700mg
- Phosphorus: 250mg

Serving Size:
- Serves 2

Cooking Time:
- 20 minutes

Lentil and Vegetable Soup

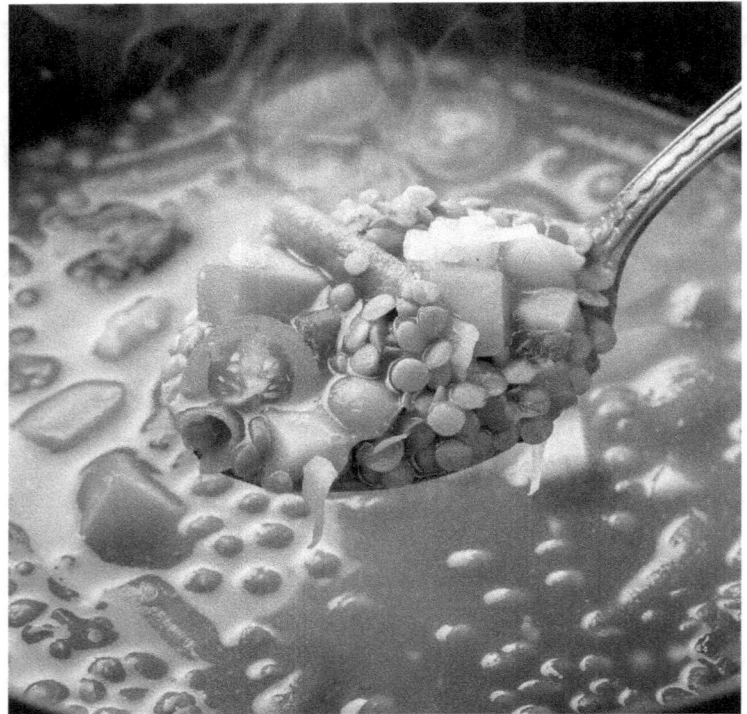

Ingredients:

- 1 cup dry lentils, rinsed
- 1 tablespoon olive oil
- 1 medium onion, chopped
- 2 cloves garlic, minced
- 2 carrots, diced
- 2 celery stalks, diced
- 1 zucchini, diced

- 1 cup spinach, chopped
- 1 teaspoon dried thyme
- 1 teaspoon dried basil
- 6 cups low-sodium vegetable broth
- 1 bay leaf
- Freshly ground black pepper to taste

Instructions:

1. In a large pot, heat the olive oil over medium heat. Add the chopped onion and cook until softened, about 5 minutes.
2. Add the minced garlic, diced carrots, and celery. Cook for another 5 minutes, stirring occasionally.
3. Add the lentils, zucchini, spinach, thyme, and basil to the pot. Stir to combine.
4. Pour in the low-sodium vegetable broth and add the bay leaf. Bring the mixture to a boil.
5. Reduce the heat to low and let the soup simmer for about 30-35 minutes, or until the lentils are tender.
6. Remove the bay leaf and season the soup with freshly ground black pepper to taste.
7. Serve hot, garnished with fresh herbs if desired.

Nutritional Information (per serving):

- Calories: 200
- Protein: 10g
- Carbohydrates: 30g
- Dietary Fiber: 12g
- Sugars: 5g

- Fat: 5g
- Sodium: 150mg
- Potassium: 400mg
- Phosphorus: 200mg

Serving Size: 1 cup

Cooking Time: 45 minutes

Quinoa and Black Bean Salad

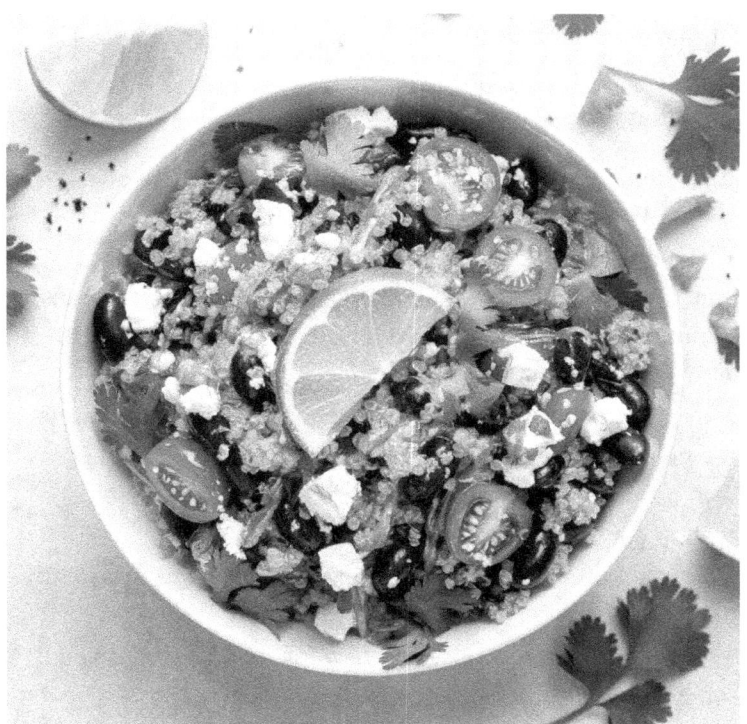

Ingredients:

- 1 cup quinoa, rinsed
- 2 cups water
- 1 can (15 ounces) black beans, rinsed and drained
- 1 red bell pepper, diced
- 1 small red onion, finely chopped
- 1 cup corn kernels (fresh or frozen)
- 1/4 cup chopped fresh cilantro

- 2 tablespoons olive oil
- 1 tablespoon lime juice
- 1 teaspoon ground cumin
- 1/2 teaspoon salt (optional)
- 1/4 teaspoon black pepper

Instructions:

1. In a medium saucepan, bring the quinoa and water to a boil. Reduce heat, cover, and simmer for about 15 minutes, or until the water is absorbed and the quinoa is tender. Fluff with a fork and let it cool slightly.
2. In a large bowl, combine the cooked quinoa, black beans, red bell pepper, red onion, corn, and cilantro.
3. In a small bowl, whisk together the olive oil, lime juice, ground cumin, salt, and black pepper.
4. Pour the dressing over the quinoa mixture and toss gently to combine.
5. Serve immediately or refrigerate for later use. This salad can be served chilled or at room temperature.

Nutritional Information (per serving):

- Calories: 250
- Protein: 8g
- Carbohydrates: 38g
- Dietary Fiber: 8g
- Sugars: 3g
- Fat: 8g
- Saturated Fat: 1g

- Sodium: 200mg (without added salt)
- Potassium: 500mg

Serving Size:
- Serves 4

Cooking Time:
- 30 minutes

Baked Cod with Steamed Broccoli

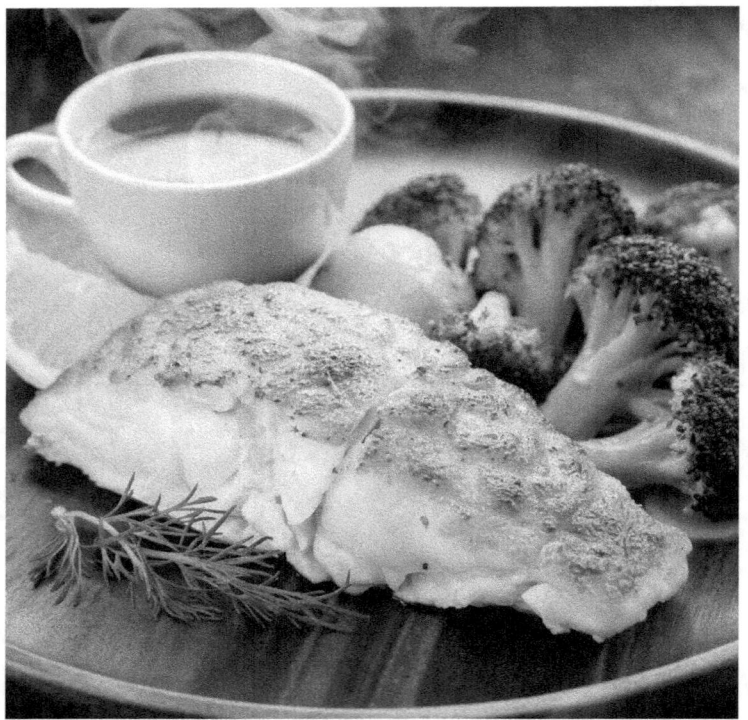

Ingredients:

- 2 cod fillets (4 ounces each)
- 1 tablespoon olive oil
- 1 teaspoon lemon juice
- 1 garlic clove, minced
- 1 teaspoon dried thyme
- Salt and pepper to taste
- 2 cups fresh broccoli florets

Instructions:

1. Preheat your oven to 400°F (200°C).
2. Place the cod fillets on a baking sheet lined with parchment paper.
3. In a small bowl, mix the olive oil, lemon juice, minced garlic, dried thyme, salt, and pepper.
4. Brush the mixture over the cod fillets.
5. Bake the cod in the preheated oven for 15-20 minutes, or until the fish flakes easily with a fork.
6. While the cod is baking, steam the broccoli florets in a steamer basket over boiling water for 5-7 minutes, until tender.
7. Serve the baked cod with the steamed broccoli on the side.

Nutritional Information:

- Calories: 220
- Protein: 28g
- Carbohydrates: 6g
- Fiber: 3g
- Fat: 10g
- Sodium: 150mg

Serving Size:

- Serves 2

Cooking Time:

- Total: 25-30 minutes

Turkey and Spinach Wrap

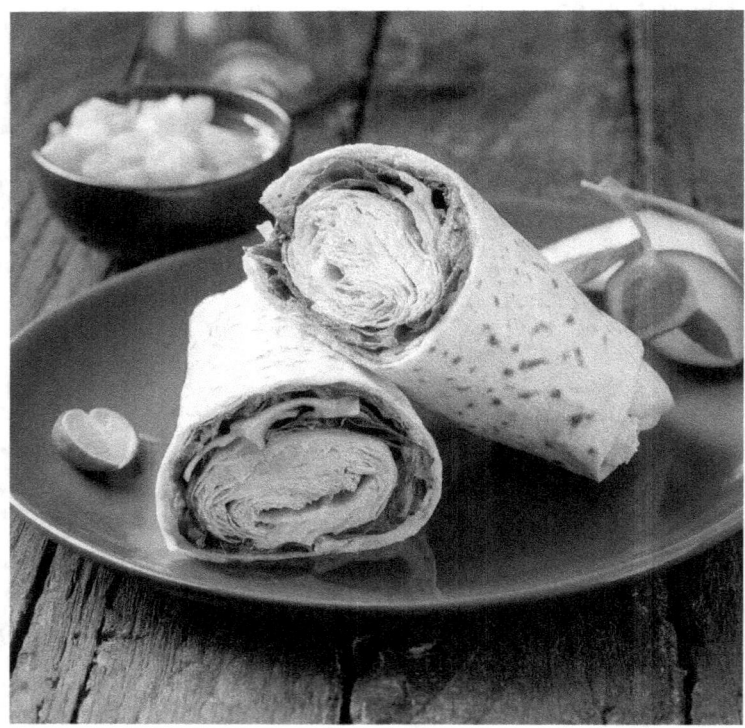

Ingredients:

- 1 whole grain tortilla (low sodium)
- 3 ounces of cooked turkey breast (sliced thin, no salt added)
- 1 cup fresh spinach leaves
- 1/4 cup shredded carrots
- 1/4 avocado, sliced

- 1 tablespoon plain Greek yogurt (optional, for added creaminess)
- 1 teaspoon lemon juice
- Freshly ground black pepper to taste

Instructions:

1. Lay the whole grain tortilla flat on a clean surface.
2. Spread the plain Greek yogurt evenly over the tortilla, if using.
3. Place the spinach leaves evenly across the tortilla.
4. Layer the turkey slices on top of the spinach.
5. Add the shredded carrots and avocado slices.
6. Sprinkle lemon juice over the ingredients and season with freshly ground black pepper.
7. Roll the tortilla tightly to enclose the filling.
8. Cut the wrap in half and serve immediately.

Nutritional Information:

- Calories: 280
- Protein: 24 grams
- Carbohydrates: 32 grams
- Dietary Fiber: 7 grams
- Total Fat: 8 grams
- Saturated Fat: 1 gram
- Sodium: 270 milligrams
- Potassium: 470 milligrams
- Phosphorus: 210 milligrams

Serving Size:
- 1 wrap

Cooking Time:
- 10 minutes

Chickpea and Avocado Sandwich

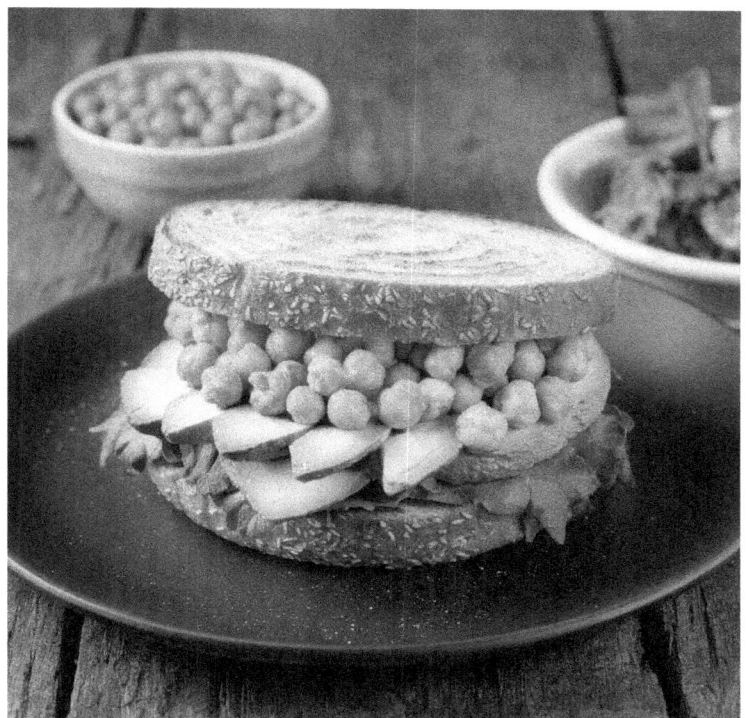

Ingredients:
- 1 ripe avocado
- 1 cup cooked chickpeas, mashed
- 2 tablespoons plain Greek yogurt
- 1 tablespoon lemon juice
- 1 teaspoon garlic powder
- Salt and pepper to taste
- 4 slices of whole-grain bread

- Fresh spinach leaves
- Sliced tomatoes

Instructions:

1. In a medium bowl, mash the ripe avocado until smooth.
2. Add the mashed chickpeas to the avocado and mix well.
3. Stir in the plain Greek yogurt, lemon juice, and garlic powder.
4. Season the mixture with salt and pepper to taste.
5. Toast the whole-grain bread slices if desired.
6. Spread the chickpea and avocado mixture evenly on two slices of bread.
7. Top with fresh spinach leaves and sliced tomatoes.
8. Place the remaining bread slices on top to form sandwiches.
9. Cut each sandwich in half and serve immediately.

Nutritional Information (per serving):

- Calories: 320
- Protein: 12g
- Carbohydrates: 38g
- Fiber: 10g
- Sugars: 5g
- Fat: 15g
- Saturated Fat: 2g
- Sodium: 180mg
- Potassium: 450mg

Serving Size: 1 sandwich

Cooking Time: 15 minutes

Roasted Vegetable and Hummus Bowl

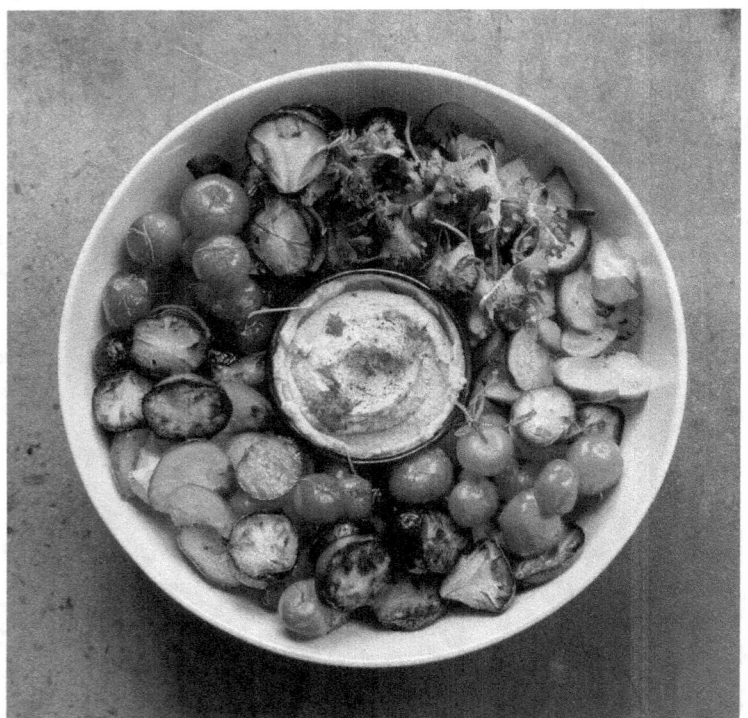

Ingredients:

- 1 cup cherry tomatoes, halved
- 1 medium zucchini, sliced
- 1 red bell pepper, chopped
- 1 yellow bell pepper, chopped
- 1 cup broccoli florets
- 2 tablespoons olive oil
- 1 teaspoon dried oregano

- Salt and pepper to taste
- 1 cup hummus (low-sodium)
- 2 cups mixed greens or cooked quinoa
- Lemon wedges for garnish

Instructions:

1. Preheat your oven to 400°F (200°C).
2. Place the cherry tomatoes, zucchini, red bell pepper, yellow bell pepper, and broccoli florets on a baking sheet.
3. Drizzle the vegetables with olive oil and sprinkle with dried oregano, salt, and pepper.
4. Toss the vegetables to ensure they are evenly coated with the oil and seasonings.
5. Roast the vegetables in the preheated oven for 20-25 minutes, or until they are tender and slightly caramelized.
6. While the vegetables are roasting, prepare your serving bowls by adding a base of mixed greens or cooked quinoa.
7. Once the vegetables are done, divide them evenly among the bowls.
8. Add a generous scoop of hummus to each bowl.
9. Garnish with lemon wedges and serve immediately.

Nutritional Information:

- Calories: 320 per serving
- Protein: 8g
- Carbohydrates: 25g
- Dietary Fiber: 10g
- Sugars: 7g

- Total Fat: 22g
- Saturated Fat: 3g
- Sodium: 240mg
- Potassium: 700mg

Serving Size:
- Makes 2 servings

Cooking Time:
- Total: 30 minutes

Cauliflower Rice Stir-Fry

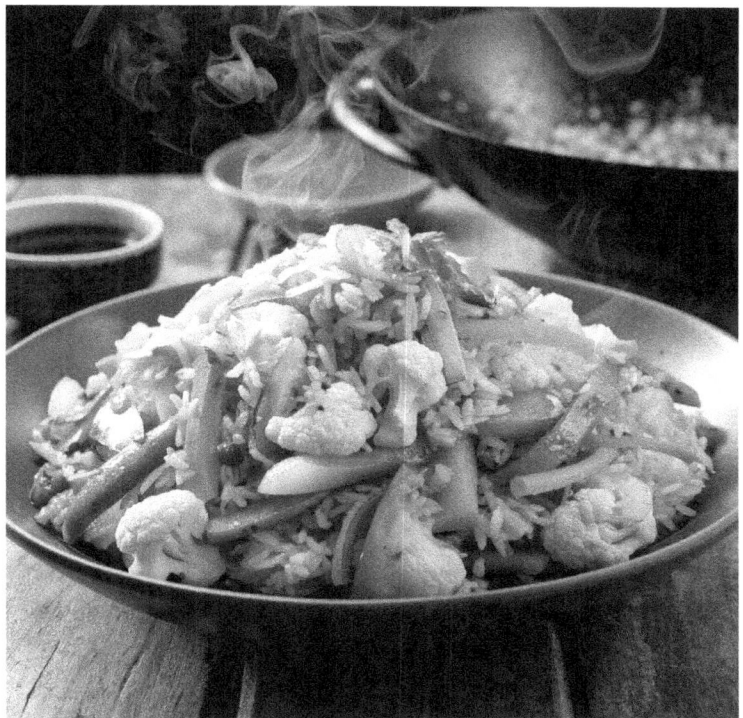

Ingredients:
- 1 small head of cauliflower, grated into rice-sized pieces
- 1 tablespoon olive oil
- 1 small onion, diced
- 1 red bell pepper, diced
- 1 cup broccoli florets
- 1 medium carrot, julienned
- 2 cloves garlic, minced

- 1 tablespoon low-sodium soy sauce
- 1 teaspoon grated fresh ginger
- 1 cup cooked chicken breast, diced
- 1 green onion, sliced
- 1 tablespoon sesame seeds (optional)

Instructions:

1. Heat the olive oil in a large skillet or wok over medium heat.
2. Add the diced onion and cook until translucent, about 3-4 minutes.
3. Add the red bell pepper, broccoli, and carrot. Stir-fry for 5-7 minutes until the vegetables are tender-crisp.
4. Add the minced garlic and grated ginger, cooking for an additional minute until fragrant.
5. Stir in the grated cauliflower rice and cook for 3-4 minutes until tender.
6. Add the low-sodium soy sauce and cooked chicken breast, stirring to combine and heat through.
7. Remove from heat and sprinkle with sliced green onion and sesame seeds, if desired.
8. Serve immediately.

Nutritional Information (per serving):

- Calories: 220
- Protein: 18g
- Carbohydrates: 14g
- Dietary Fiber: 6g

- Sugars: 5g
- Fat: 10g
- Saturated Fat: 1.5g
- Sodium: 240mg
- Potassium: 550mg

Serving Size: 1 cup

Cooking Time: 20 minutes

Mediterranean Tuna Salad

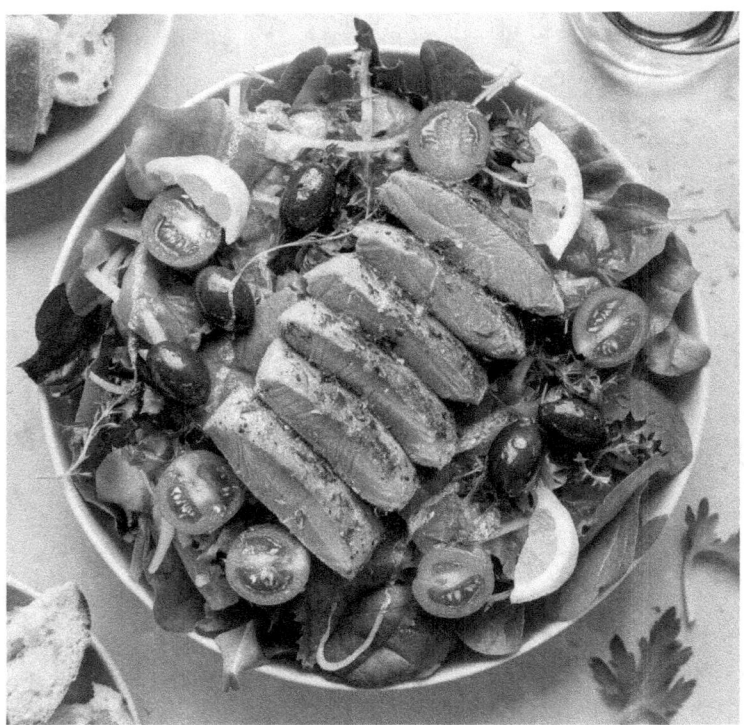

Ingredients:

- 1 can (5 ounces) low-sodium tuna, drained
- 1 cup cherry tomatoes, halved
- 1/2 cup cucumber, diced
- 1/4 cup red onion, finely chopped
- 1/4 cup Kalamata olives, pitted and sliced
- 1/4 cup crumbled feta cheese
- 2 tablespoons olive oil

- 1 tablespoon lemon juice
- 1 teaspoon dried oregano
- Salt and pepper to taste
- 4 cups mixed greens (spinach, arugula, or lettuce)

Instructions:

1. In a large bowl, combine the tuna, cherry tomatoes, cucumber, red onion, olives, and feta cheese.
2. In a small bowl, whisk together the olive oil, lemon juice, oregano, salt, and pepper to create the dressing.
3. Pour the dressing over the tuna mixture and gently toss to combine.
4. Serve the tuna salad over a bed of mixed greens.

Nutritional Information (per serving):

- Calories: 250
- Protein: 18g
- Carbohydrates: 6g
- Dietary Fiber: 2g
- Total Sugars: 2g
- Total Fat: 16g
- Saturated Fat: 4g
- Sodium: 350mg
- Potassium: 400mg

Serving Size: 1 cup tuna salad over 1 cup mixed greens

Cooking Time: 15 minutes

Zucchini Noodles with Pesto and Cherry Tomatoes

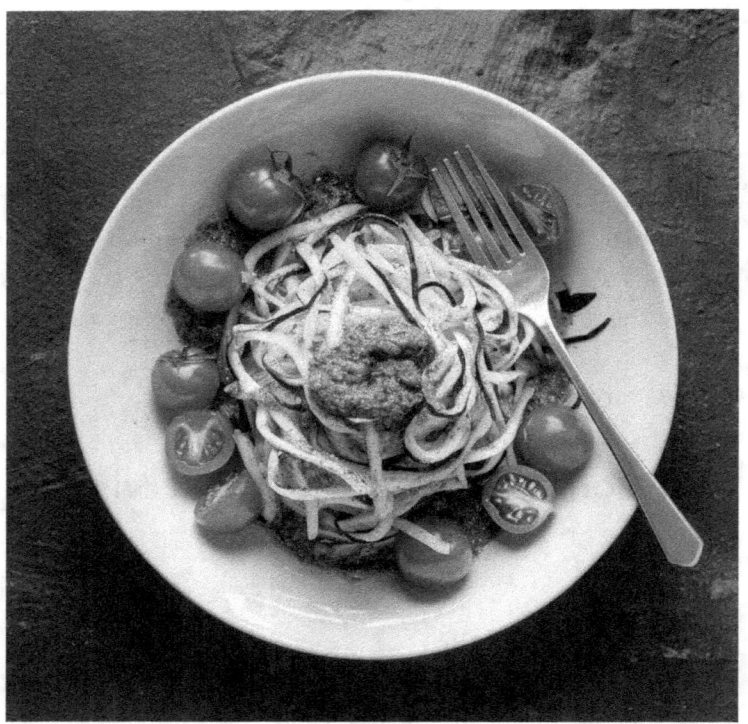

Ingredients

- 2 medium zucchinis, spiralized
- 1 cup cherry tomatoes, halved
- 1/4 cup fresh basil leaves
- 1/4 cup pine nuts, toasted
- 1/4 cup grated Parmesan cheese
- 1 clove garlic

- 1/4 cup extra virgin olive oil
- Salt and pepper to taste

Instructions

1. Using a spiralizer, create zucchini noodles and set them aside.
2. In a food processor, combine the basil leaves, pine nuts, Parmesan cheese, and garlic. Pulse until finely chopped.
3. With the food processor running, slowly add the olive oil until the pesto reaches a smooth consistency. Season with salt and pepper to taste.
4. In a large bowl, toss the zucchini noodles with the prepared pesto until evenly coated.
5. Gently fold in the cherry tomatoes.
6. Serve immediately or chill in the refrigerator for up to 2 hours before serving.

Nutritional Information (per serving)

- Calories: 220
- Protein: 4g
- Carbohydrates: 8g
- Dietary Fiber: 2g
- Total Sugars: 5g
- Fat: 20g
- Saturated Fat: 3g
- Sodium: 140mg
- Potassium: 380mg
- Phosphorus: 90mg

Serving Size
- 2 servings

Cooking Time
- 20 minutes

Chapter 3: Dinner Choices

Herb-Crusted Salmon with Asparagus

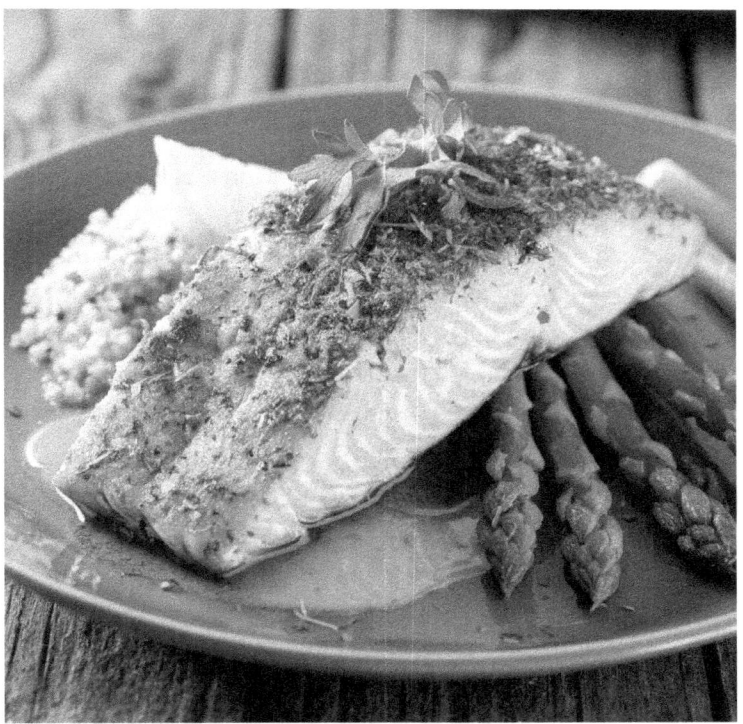

Ingredient:

- 4 salmon fillets (about 6 ounces each)
- 1 tablespoon olive oil
- 2 cloves garlic, minced
- 1 teaspoon dried thyme

- 1 teaspoon dried rosemary
- 1 teaspoon dried parsley
- 1/2 teaspoon black pepper
- 1/4 teaspoon salt (optional, or low-sodium substitute)
- 1 lemon, thinly sliced
- 1 bunch asparagus, trimmed

Instructions:

1. Preheat your oven to 400°F (200°C). Line a baking sheet with parchment paper.
2. In a small bowl, mix together the olive oil, minced garlic, thyme, rosemary, parsley, black pepper, and salt.
3. Place the salmon fillets on the prepared baking sheet. Rub the herb mixture evenly over the top of each fillet.
4. Arrange the lemon slices on top of the salmon fillets.
5. Place the asparagus spears around the salmon on the baking sheet. Drizzle with a little extra olive oil if desired.
6. Bake in the preheated oven for 15-20 minutes, or until the salmon is cooked through and flakes easily with a fork, and the asparagus is tender.
7. Serve immediately, garnished with additional lemon slices if desired.

Nutritional Information (per serving):

- Calories: 300
- Protein: 30g
- Carbohydrates: 4g
- Dietary Fiber: 2g

- Sugars: 1g
- Fat: 18g
- Saturated Fat: 3g
- Sodium: 180mg
- Potassium: 850mg
- Phosphorus: 300mg

Serving Size: 1 salmon fillet with a portion of asparagus

Cooking Time: 30 minutes (including preparation and cooking)

Stuffed Bell Peppers with Ground Turkey

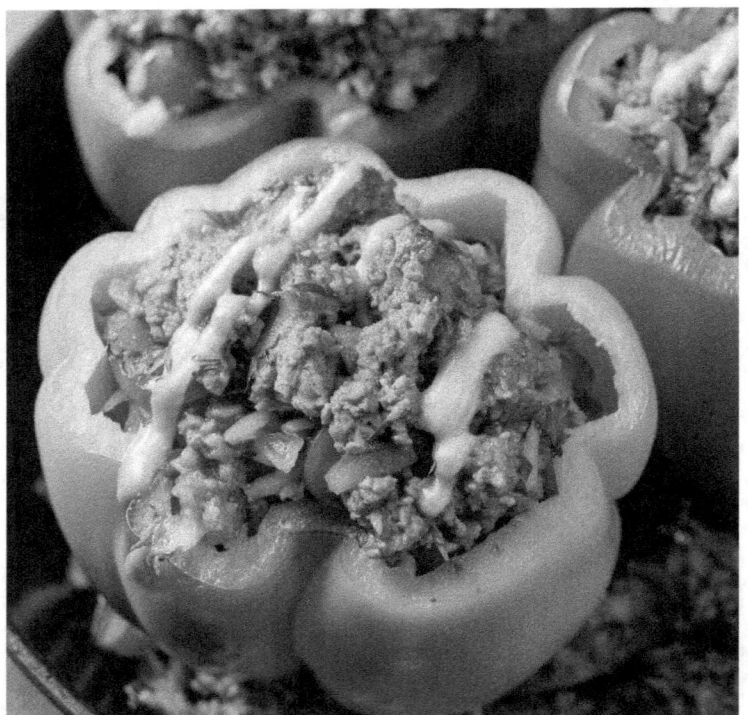

Ingredient:

- 4 large bell peppers, any color
- 1 lb ground turkey
- 1 small onion, finely chopped
- 2 cloves garlic, minced
- 1 cup cooked quinoa
- 1 cup low-sodium tomato sauce
- 1 tsp dried oregano

- 1 tsp dried basil
- Salt and pepper to taste
- 1 cup shredded low-fat mozzarella cheese

Instructions:
1. Preheat your oven to 375°F (190°C).
2. Cut the tops off the bell peppers and remove the seeds and membranes. Set aside.
3. In a large skillet, cook the ground turkey over medium heat until browned. Drain any excess fat.
4. Add the chopped onion and minced garlic to the skillet. Cook until the onion is translucent.
5. Stir in the cooked quinoa, tomato sauce, oregano, basil, salt, and pepper. Mix well and cook for another 5 minutes.
6. Stuff each bell pepper with the turkey and quinoa mixture, packing it down gently.
7. Place the stuffed peppers in a baking dish and top each with shredded mozzarella cheese.
8. Cover the dish with aluminum foil and bake for 30 minutes.
9. Remove the foil and bake for an additional 10-15 minutes, or until the peppers are tender and the cheese is melted and bubbly.

Nutritional Information:
- Calories: 280 per serving
- Protein: 25g
- Carbohydrates: 20g

- Dietary Fiber: 5g
- Sugars: 6g
- Fat: 10g
- Saturated Fat: 4g
- Sodium: 320mg
- Potassium: 650mg
- Phosphorus: 260mg

Serving Size: 1 stuffed pepper

Cooking Time: 50-60 minutes

Baked Chicken with Rosemary and Sweet Potatoes

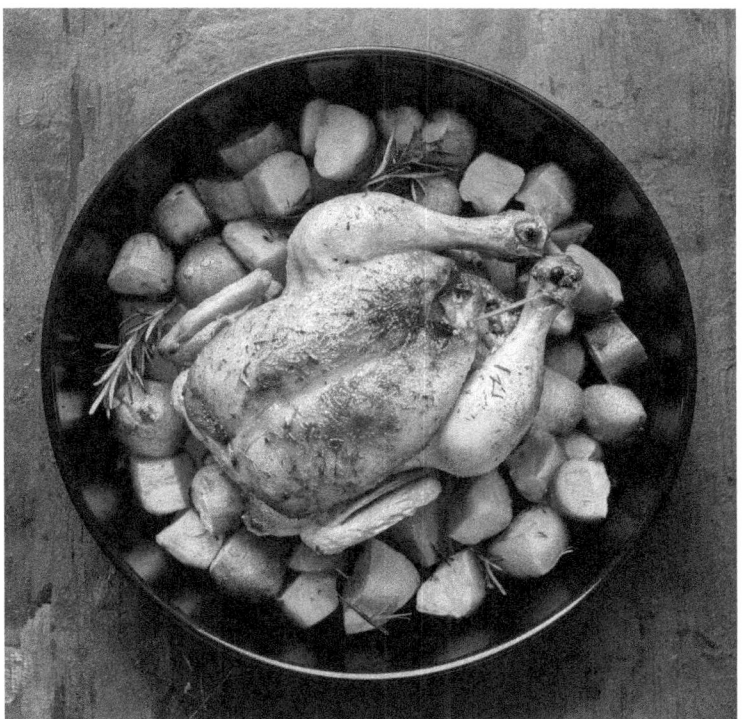

Ingredients:
- 4 boneless, skinless chicken breasts
- 2 large sweet potatoes, peeled and cut into cubes
- 2 tablespoons olive oil
- 2 teaspoons dried rosemary
- 1 teaspoon garlic powder
- 1 teaspoon paprika

- Salt and pepper to taste
- Fresh parsley for garnish (optional)

Instructions:

1. Preheat your oven to 400°F (200°C).
2. In a large bowl, toss the sweet potatoes with 1 tablespoon of olive oil, 1 teaspoon of rosemary, garlic powder, paprika, salt, and pepper until evenly coated.
3. Spread the sweet potatoes in a single layer on a baking sheet lined with parchment paper.
4. In the same bowl, coat the chicken breasts with the remaining olive oil and rosemary, then season with salt and pepper.
5. Place the chicken breasts on the baking sheet alongside the sweet potatoes.
6. Bake in the preheated oven for 25-30 minutes, or until the chicken is cooked through and the sweet potatoes are tender.
7. Garnish with fresh parsley before serving, if desired.

Nutritional Information:

- Calories: 350 per serving
- Protein: 30 grams
- Carbohydrates: 25 grams
- Dietary Fiber: 4 grams
- Sugars: 6 grams
- Fat: 12 grams
- Saturated Fat: 2 grams

- Sodium: 180 milligrams
- Potassium: 750 milligrams

Serving Size:
- Serves 4

Cooking Time:
- Preparation Time: 15 minutes
- Cooking Time: 25-30 minutes

Spinach and Ricotta Stuffed Portobello Mushrooms

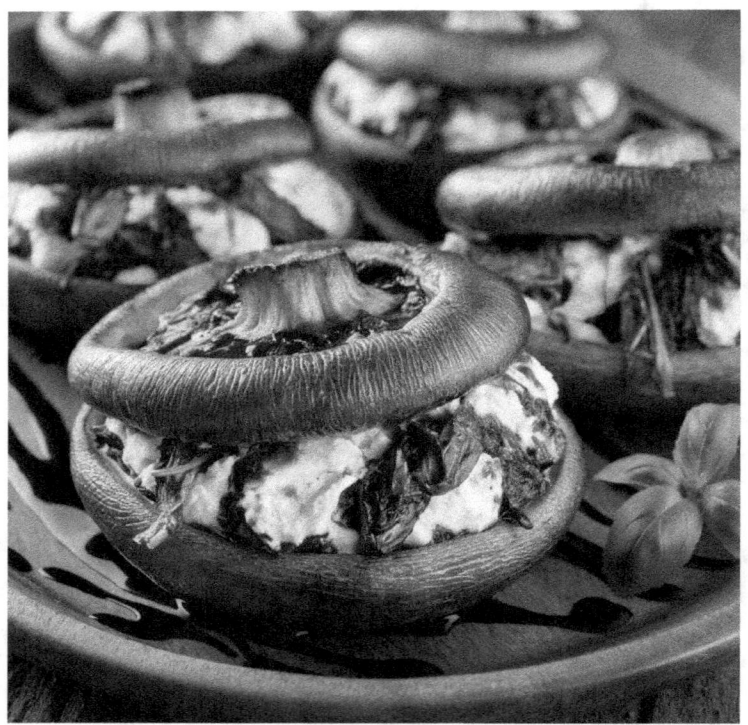

Ingredients:

- 4 large portobello mushrooms, stems removed
- 1 cup ricotta cheese
- 2 cups fresh spinach, chopped
- 1 clove garlic, minced
- 1/4 cup grated Parmesan cheese
- 2 tablespoons olive oil

- Salt and pepper to taste (use low sodium salt for kidney health)

Instructions:

1. Preheat your oven to 375°F (190°C).
2. In a skillet, heat one tablespoon of olive oil over medium heat. Add garlic and sauté until fragrant, about 1 minute.
3. Add spinach to the skillet and cook until wilted, about 3-4 minutes. Remove from heat.
4. In a bowl, combine the sautéed spinach, ricotta cheese, and half of the Parmesan cheese. Season with salt and pepper.
5. Brush the mushroom caps with the remaining olive oil and place them on a baking sheet.
6. Divide the spinach and ricotta mixture evenly among the mushroom caps, stuffing them generously.
7. Sprinkle the remaining Parmesan cheese over the stuffed mushrooms.
8. Bake in the preheated oven until the mushrooms are tender and the cheese is golden, about 20-25 minutes.

Nutritional Information:

- Calories: 200
- Carbohydrates: 6g
- Protein: 12g
- Fat: 15g
- Sodium: 180mg
- Fiber: 2g

Serving Size:
- 1 stuffed mushroom per serving

Cooking Time:
- Total preparation and cooking time: 35 minutes

Beef and Broccoli Stir-Fry

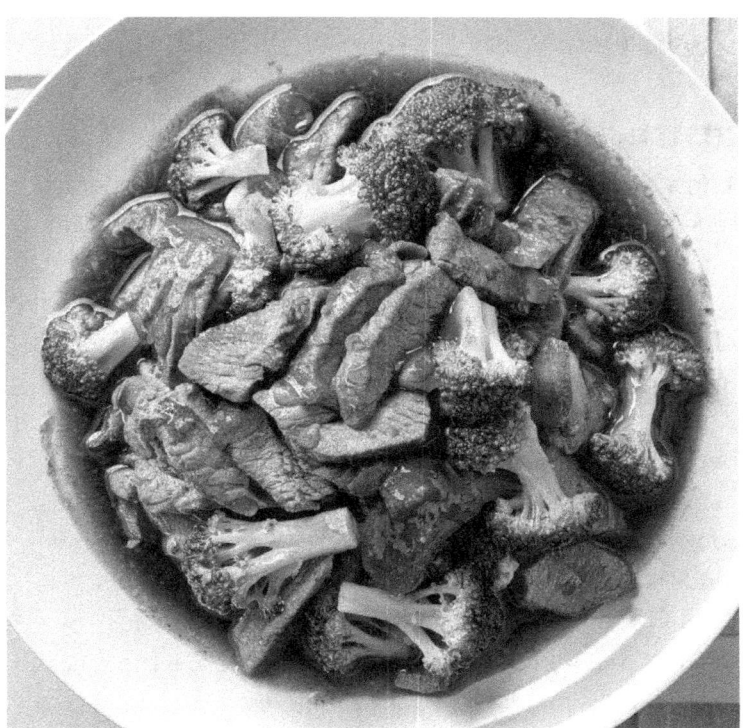

Ingredient:
- 1 pound lean beef, thinly sliced
- 4 cups broccoli florets
- 1 tablespoon olive oil
- 2 cloves garlic, minced
- 1/2 cup low-sodium beef broth
- 1 tablespoon cornstarch
- 2 tablespoons low-sodium soy sauce

- 1 tablespoon oyster sauce
- 1 teaspoon sesame oil
- Fresh ginger, a 1-inch piece grated

Instructions:

1. In a small bowl, mix the beef broth, soy sauce, oyster sauce, cornstarch, and sesame oil until well combined. Set the sauce aside.
2. Heat the olive oil in a large skillet over medium-high heat. Add the garlic and ginger, sautéing for about 30 seconds until fragrant.
3. Add the beef to the skillet and cook until it is browned and nearly cooked through, approximately 3-4 minutes.
4. Incorporate the broccoli florets, stirring frequently, and cook for an additional 4-5 minutes until the vegetables are tender but still crisp.
5. Reduce the heat to medium-low and pour the sauce over the beef and broccoli. Stir well to coat and allow the sauce to thicken as it simmers for about 2 minutes.
6. Remove from heat and serve warm.

Nutritional Information:

- Calories: 250 per serving
- Protein: 26g
- Carbohydrates: 15g
- Fat: 10g
- Sodium: 320mg
- Fiber: 3g

Serving Size: Serves 4

Cooking Time: Approximately 20 minutes

Lemon Garlic Shrimp with Quinoa

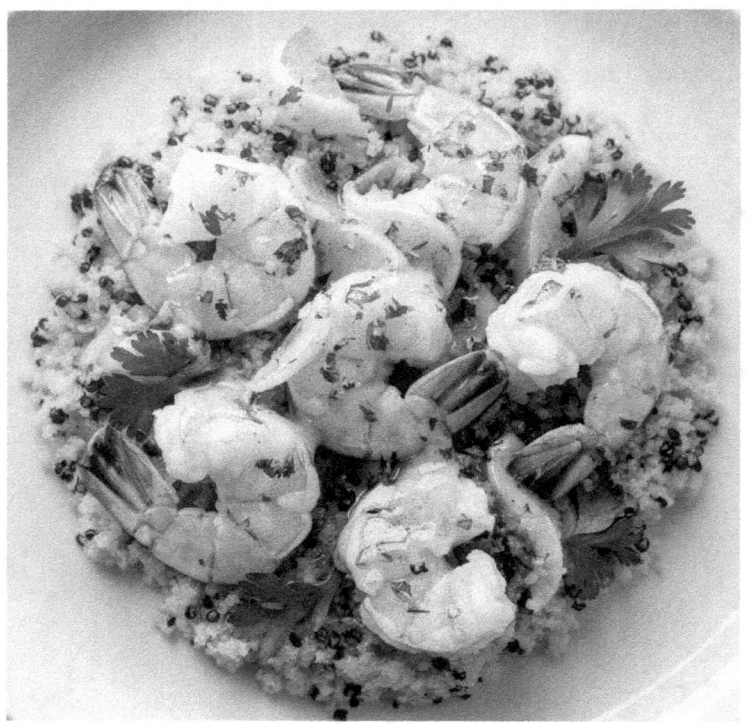

Ingredients

- 1 pound of large shrimp, peeled and deveined
- 2 tablespoons of olive oil
- Juice and zest of 1 lemon
- 3 cloves of garlic, minced
- 1 teaspoon of black pepper
- 1 cup of quinoa
- 2 cups of low-sodium vegetable broth

- 1/4 cup of fresh parsley, chopped

Instructions

1. Rinse the quinoa thoroughly under cold running water. In a medium saucepan, bring the low-sodium vegetable broth to a boil. Add the quinoa, reduce heat to low, cover, and simmer for 15-20 minutes or until all the liquid is absorbed.
2. While the quinoa is cooking, heat olive oil in a large skillet over medium heat. Add the minced garlic and sauté for about 1 minute, until fragrant.
3. Add the shrimp to the skillet, and sprinkle with black pepper and half of the lemon zest. Cook for 2-3 minutes on each side or until the shrimp turn pink and are cooked through.
4. Once the shrimp are done, stir in the lemon juice and remove from heat.
5. Fluff the cooked quinoa with a fork and mix in the remaining lemon zest and chopped parsley.
6. Serve the shrimp over the quinoa.

Nutritional Information

- Calories: 350 per serving
- Protein: 28 grams
- Carbohydrates: 35 grams
- Fat: 10 grams
- Sodium: 180 mg
- Potassium: 470 mg
- Phosphorus: 290 mg

Serving Size
- This recipe serves 4.

Cooking Time
- Preparation time: 10 minutes
- Cooking time: 30 minutes
- Total time: 40 minutes

Eggplant Parmesan (Baked)

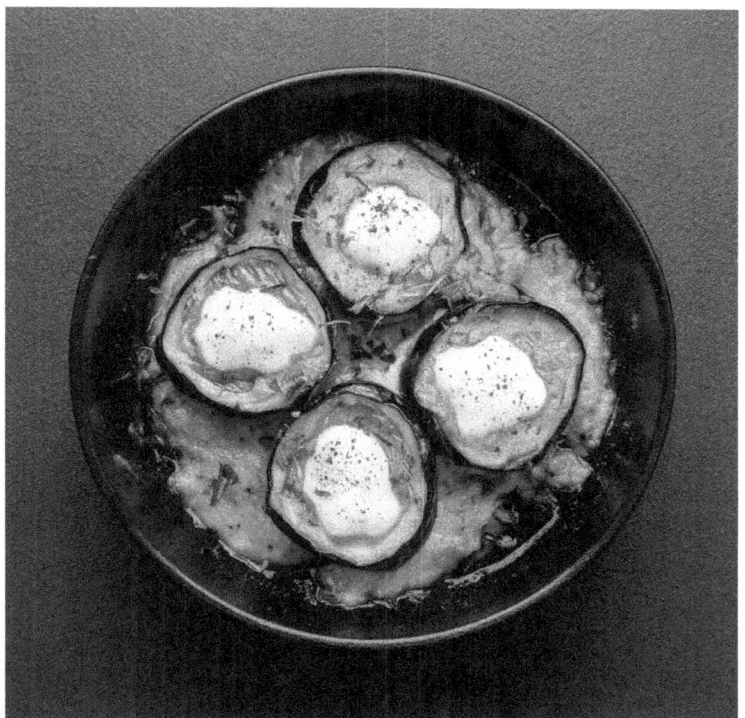

Ingredients:

- Eggplant, sliced into rounds
- Low-sodium marinara sauce
- Shredded mozzarella cheese (low-fat)
- Grated Parmesan cheese (low-fat)
- Olive oil
- Ground black pepper
- Fresh basil leaves for garnish

- Egg substitute for coating
- Whole wheat or almond flour for breading
- Cooking spray

Instructions:

1. Preheat the oven to 375°F (190°C).
2. Lightly coat the sliced eggplant with olive oil and season with ground black pepper.
3. Dip the seasoned eggplant slices first in egg substitute, then coat with flour.
4. Arrange the coated eggplant slices on a baking sheet lined with parchment paper and lightly coated with cooking spray.
5. Bake for 25 minutes, flipping halfway through, until the eggplant is golden and tender.
6. In a baking dish, layer the baked eggplant slices with marinara sauce and sprinkle with mozzarella and Parmesan cheeses.
7. Bake in the oven for an additional 20 minutes, or until the cheese is bubbly and golden.
8. Garnish with fresh basil leaves before serving.

Nutritional Information (per serving):

- Calories: Approximately 200
- Carbohydrates: 18g
- Protein: 12g
- Fat: 10g
- Sodium: 200mg
- Potassium: 450mg

- Phosphorus: 150mg

Serving Size:
- This recipe serves 4 individuals.

Cooking Time:
- Preparation time: 15 minutes
- Cooking time: 45 minutes
- Total time: 60 minutes

Grilled Tofu with Steamed Vegetables

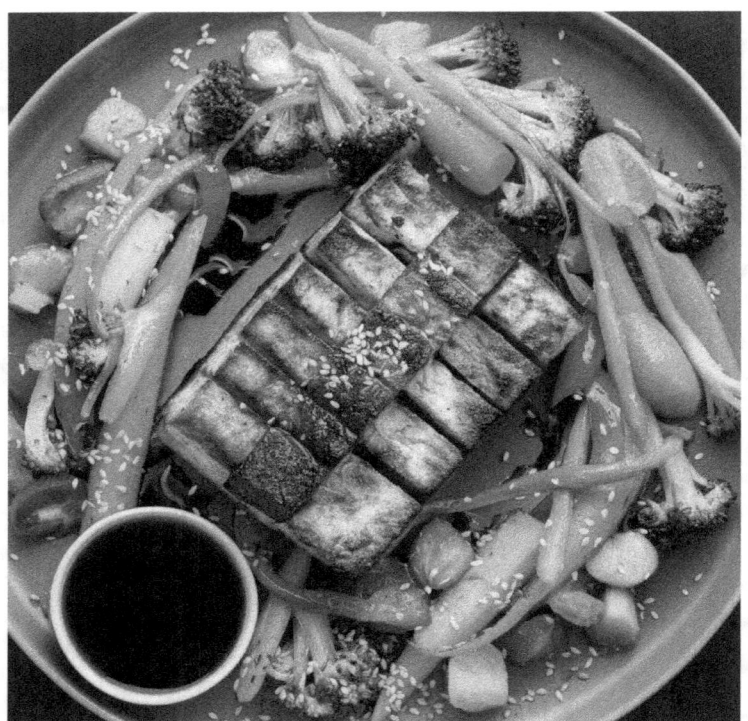

Ingredients

- 14 oz firm tofu, drained and pressed
- 1 tablespoon olive oil
- 1/2 teaspoon garlic powder
- 1/2 teaspoon onion powder
- Salt (optional) and pepper to taste
- 2 cups broccoli florets
- 1 cup sliced carrots

- 1 cup bell pepper strips
- Fresh lemon juice (for serving)

Instructions

1. Preheat your grill or grill pan over medium heat.
2. Cut the tofu into 1/2 inch thick slices. Brush each slice with olive oil and season with garlic powder, onion powder, and a little salt and pepper if desired.
3. Place tofu slices on the grill and cook for about 4-5 minutes on each side or until they have nice grill marks and are heated through.
4. While the tofu grills, steam the broccoli, carrots, and bell peppers until they are tender but still crisp, about 5-7 minutes.
5. Serve the grilled tofu with the steamed vegetables on the side. Squeeze fresh lemon juice over the tofu and vegetables for added flavor.

Nutritional Information

- Calories: 200
- Protein: 15g
- Carbohydrates: 14g
- Fiber: 5g
- Sodium: 60mg (varies if salt is added)
- Fat: 10g

Serving Size

- Serves 4

Cooking Time
- Total Time: 20 minutes

Spaghetti Squash with Turkey Marinara

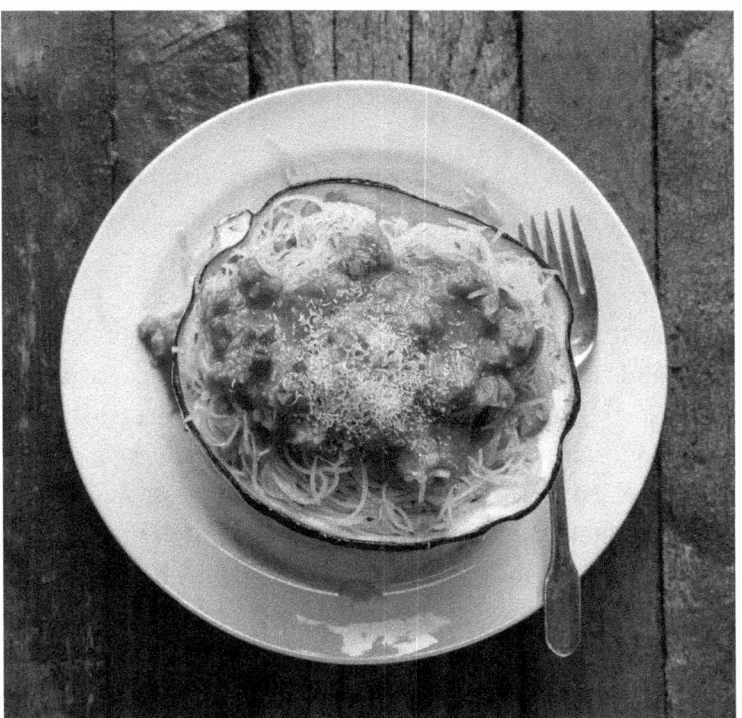

Ingredients

- 1 large spaghetti squash (about 2 pounds)
- 1 tablespoon olive oil
- 1 pound ground turkey
- 1/2 cup chopped onion
- 2 garlic cloves, minced
- 1 can (28 ounces) no-salt-added crushed tomatoes
- 1 teaspoon dried basil

- 1 teaspoon dried oregano
- Salt and pepper to taste (optional)
- Fresh basil leaves, for garnish

Instructions

1. Preheat oven to 400°F (200°C). Halve the spaghetti squash lengthwise and scoop out the seeds. Place squash halves cut-side down on a baking sheet and roast for 40 minutes, or until tender.
2. While the squash is roasting, heat olive oil in a large skillet over medium heat. Add the ground turkey, onion, and garlic. Cook, stirring to crumble the turkey, until it is no longer pink.
3. Stir in the crushed tomatoes, dried basil, and oregano. Bring to a simmer and cook for about 20 minutes, allowing flavors to meld. Season with salt and pepper if desired.
4. Once the squash is cooked, let it cool slightly before using a fork to scrape the inside, creating spaghetti-like strands.
5. To serve, place a portion of the spaghetti squash on a plate and top with the turkey marinara. Garnish with fresh basil leaves.

Nutritional Information

- Calories: 290
- Protein: 27g
- Fat: 14g
- Carbohydrates: 18g
- Fiber: 4g
- Sodium: 80mg

Serving Size

- 1 cup of cooked spaghetti squash topped with 3/4 cup of turkey marinara

Cooking Time

- Prep time: 10 minutes
- Cook time: 60 minutes
- Total time: 70 minutes

Vegetable and Lentil Stew

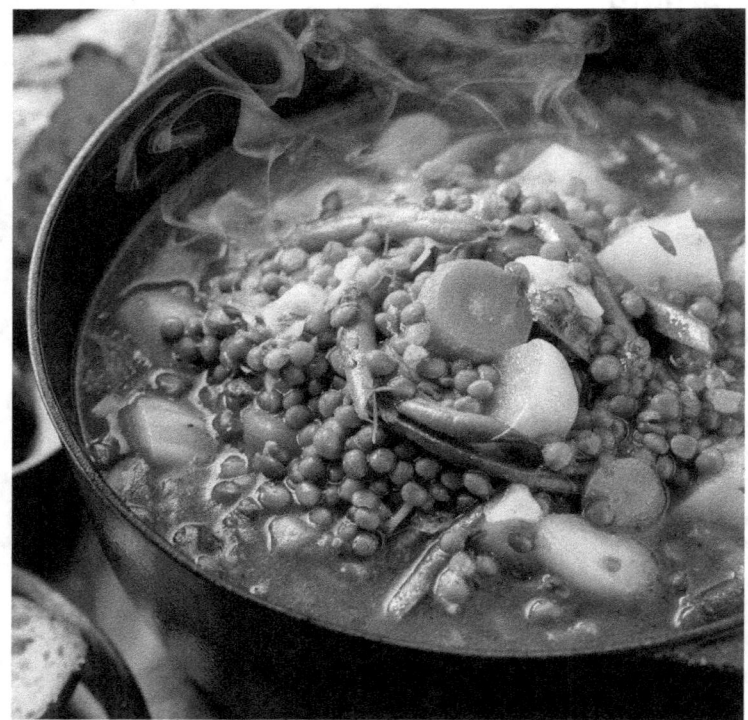

Ingredients

- 1 tablespoon olive oil
- 1 large onion, diced
- 2 cloves garlic, minced
- 2 carrots, peeled and diced
- 2 stalks celery, diced
- 1 red bell pepper, diced
- 1 zucchini, diced

- 1 cup dried lentils, rinsed
- 1 teaspoon dried thyme
- 1 teaspoon dried rosemary
- 4 cups low-sodium vegetable broth
- 2 cups water
- Salt and pepper to taste (use sparingly)
- 2 cups chopped kale

Instructions

1. Heat the olive oil in a large pot over medium heat. Add the onion and garlic and sauté until the onion is translucent.
2. Add the carrots, celery, bell pepper, and zucchini to the pot and cook for about 5 minutes, until they begin to soften.
3. Stir in the lentils, thyme, and rosemary, then pour in the vegetable broth and water.
4. Bring the mixture to a boil, then reduce the heat and let it simmer for about 25 minutes, or until the lentils are tender.
5. Add the kale and continue to simmer for another 5 minutes.
6. Season with salt and pepper to taste, remembering to keep sodium intake minimal.
7. Serve hot.

Nutritional Information (per serving)

- Calories: 220
- Protein: 14 g
- Carbohydrates: 35 g
- Fiber: 15 g

- Sodium: 70 mg
- Potassium: 600 mg
- Phosphorus: 150 mg

Serving Size
- Makes 6 servings

Cooking Time
- Prep time: 10 minutes
- Cook time: 40 minutes
- Total time: 50 minutes

Chapter 4: Snacks and Sides

Cucumber and Hummus Bites

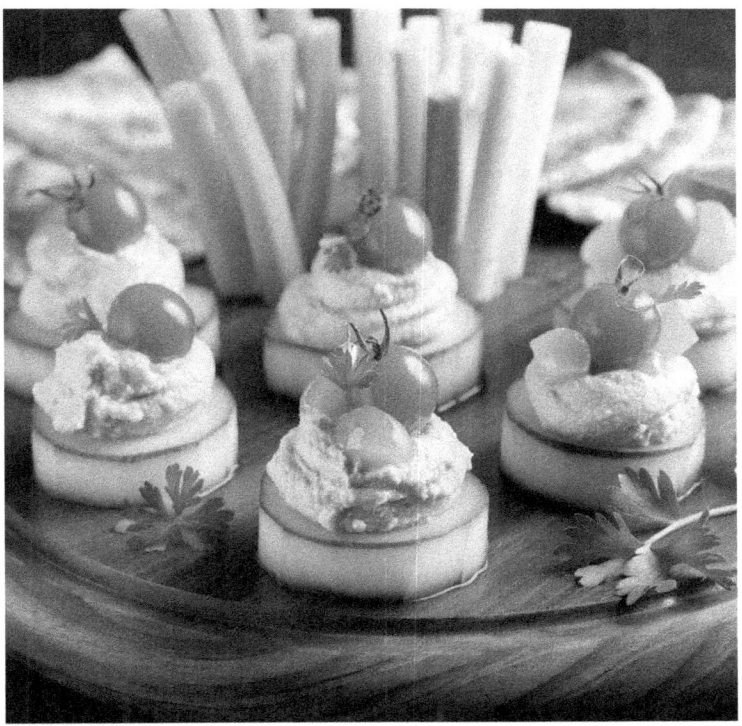

Ingredient:
- 1 large cucumber
- 1 cup low-sodium, low-phosphorus hummus
- Paprika for garnish
- Fresh parsley, finely chopped (optional for garnish)

Instructions:

1. Wash the cucumber thoroughly and slice it into rounds about 1/4 inch thick.
2. Spoon a small amount of hummus on each cucumber slice.
3. Sprinkle a dash of paprika over the hummus for added flavor.
4. If desired, top each bite with a sprinkle of finely chopped fresh parsley for a fresh, herbal touch.

Nutritional Information:

- Calories: Approximately 35 calories per serving
- Protein: 2 grams per serving
- Sodium: Less than 50 mg per serving
- Potassium: Approximately 49 mg per serving
- Phosphorus: Less than 12 mg per serving

Serving Size:

- 1 bite (adjust number of servings based on personal meal plan requirements)

Cooking Time:

- Prep Time: 10 minutes
- Total Time: 10 minutes

Baked Kale Chips

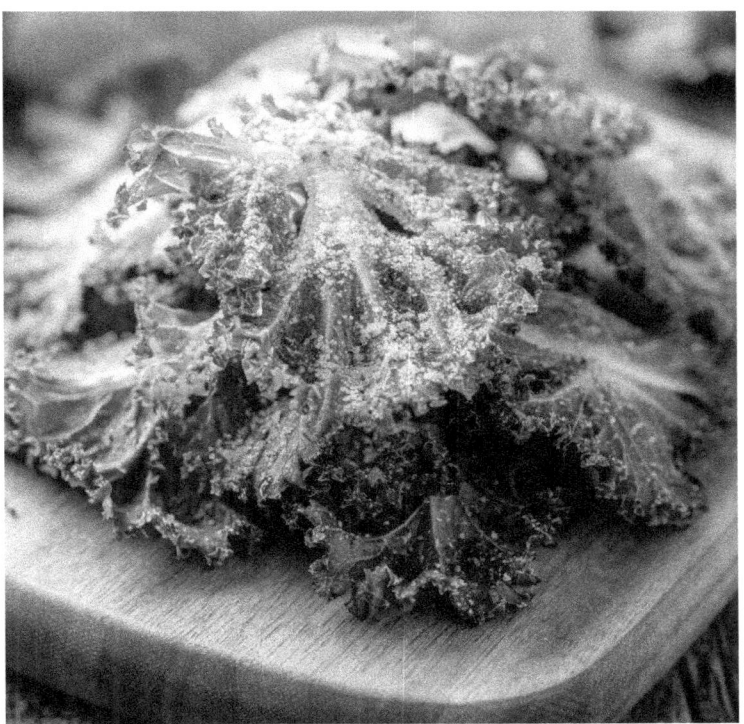

Ingredient:

- 1 bunch of fresh kale, washed and dried
- 1 tablespoon olive oil
- 1/4 teaspoon salt (optional, can be omitted or reduced for lower sodium needs)

Instructions:

1. Preheat your oven to 275 degrees Fahrenheit.

2. Remove the stems and tough center ribs from the kale leaves, then tear the leaves into bite-size pieces.
3. In a large bowl, gently toss the kale pieces with olive oil and salt (if using) until evenly coated.
4. Spread the kale in a single layer on a baking sheet lined with parchment paper.
5. Bake in the preheated oven for about 20 minutes, turning the leaves halfway through, until crisp and lightly browned. Watch carefully to avoid over-baking.

Nutritional Information:
- Calories: 58 per serving
- Carbohydrates: 7g
- Protein: 2g
- Fat: 3g
- Sodium: 99mg (without added salt)

Serving Size:
- Serves 4

Cooking Time:
- Prep Time: 10 minutes
- Cook Time: 20 minutes

Conclusion

As we reach the conclusion of the "Diabetic Renal Diet Cookbook for Beginners 2024," it's important to reflect on the journey we've embarked upon together. This cookbook was crafted with the dual purpose of simplifying the dietary management of diabetes and kidney disease and enriching your life with culinary delights that cater to these specific health needs. The recipes and guidelines provided have been meticulously designed to assist you in maintaining a balanced and nutritious diet that supports your health conditions without sacrificing flavor or enjoyment.

The path to managing diabetes and kidney disease through diet can be challenging, but it is also incredibly rewarding. This cookbook has aimed to demystify the process, providing you with the tools and knowledge needed to prepare meals that are both beneficial and enjoyable. By incorporating these recipes into your daily life, you have taken significant steps towards stabilizing blood sugar levels, protecting kidney function, and enhancing your overall well-being.

Throughout this book, we have emphasized the importance of understanding the nutritional content of your meals, the impact of various foods on your health, and the methods of preparing dishes that are safe and healthful. The guidance on meal planning and preparation techniques has been included to make your dietary routine as straightforward and effective as possible. These elements are crucial as they empower you to make informed decisions about your diet every day.

The feedback loop between your dietary choices and your health is ongoing, and this cookbook serves as a resource you can continually refer to. It's designed to grow with you as you advance in your dietary management journey. You may find yourself returning to different sections for recipe inspiration or to revisit nutritional advice as your health needs evolve.

Encouragement is key in maintaining the motivation needed for a lifestyle change. Remember, every meal prepared using this guide is a step towards better health. Celebrate the small victories, whether it's noticing improvements in your health metrics, feeling more energetic, or simply enjoying a meal that tastes great and is good for you. These positive reinforcements are essential for long-term success.

For further support, the book directs you to resources where you can find additional information, connect with communities of individuals facing similar challenges, and seek professional advice when needed. Leveraging these resources can enhance your ability to manage your health conditions effectively and stay updated on the latest in diabetes and renal health care.

In conclusion, the "Diabetic Renal Diet Cookbook for Beginners 2024" is not just a collection of recipes—it's a companion in your journey towards health and vitality. Continue to use it as a guide, a source of inspiration, and a tool for transformation. With every dish you prepare, you're taking control of your health, one delicious bite at a time. Your commitment to following this path is commendable, and the strides you make in managing your diabetes and kidney health through diet are worth celebrating.

www.ingramcontent.com/pod-product-compliance
Lightning Source LLC
Chambersburg PA
CBHW071523220526
45472CB00003B/1128